ALTERNATIVE
MATERNITY

NICKY WESSON

ILLUSTRATED BY
DAVID RAITT

An OPTIMA book

© Nicky Wesson, 1989

First published in 1989 by
Macdonald Optima, a division of
Macdonald & Co. (Publishers) Ltd

A member of Maxwell Pergamon Publishing Corporation plc

British Library Cataloguing in Publication Data

Wesson, Nicky
Alternative maternity
1. Pregnant women. Alternative
methods
I. Title
618.2′06

ISBN 0-356-15412-2

Macdonald & Co. (Publishers) Ltd
66-73 Shoe Lane
London EC4P 4AB

Typeset in Century Schoolbook by Leaper & Gard, Bristol

Printed and bound in Great Britain
by The Guernsey Press Co. Ltd., Guernsey, Channel Islands.

CONTENTS

PREFACE

When my first child was born eleven years ago, I was completely wedded to the medical model. It had simply never occurred to me to do anything other than go to a doctor when ill. My daughter Alicia was born in hospital and returned there five weeks later with a problem which remained undiagnosed. She had severe colic, was frequently ill, and consumed pints of antibiotics. She had a couple of operations as a result of constant ear infections and, understandably, was not always a happy child. My next child, Duncan, was born after a complicated labour and an emergency caesarean section. He too had constant ear infections, eczema and, we eventually discovered, an allergy to milk, wheat and eggs. Hospital care, a very restricted diet, and drugs kept both Alicia and Duncan reasonably well, but not without difficulties, side-effects and a feeling of unease at having such young children on constant medication.

In 1984, when our third child, Alastair, was a few months old, I attended a conference that was to revolutionise our lives. The topic was alternative medicine for pregnancy, labour and babies, and it covered acupuncture, homeopathy, herbalism and osteopathy. I knew at once that this might offer solutions to the problems we were still struggling with. Alastair was proving more severely allergic; we even had to drop out of a double-blind trial testing breastfed babies who had eczema because he reacted so badly to allergens in my breast milk whenever I had egg and milk.

Not without misgivings, I took him to the acupuncturist, Adrian Stoddart, who had given the lecture. He applied acupressure to him and, literally overnight his food sensitivity decreased. Due partly to luck and partly to my newly gained knowledge which I enthusiastically put into practice, both Alastair and his younger sister Octavia have never taken an antibiotic.

Cranial osteopathy on the two older children who both had instrumental deliveries has put a stop to the ear infections and means they are far happier. It has even obviated the need for my eleven year old to have four of her adult teeth removed and wear a brace. Octavia, now two, was treated for colic soon after birth and has since remained sunny and relaxed. Having osteopathic treatment myself before the birth meant that she almost shot out, in sharp contrast to my difficult labours previously.

Acupuncture has improved the health of myself and my children enormously, we use herbs to treat infection, and have used homeopathy and hypnotherapy on occasion with success. Through recommending these alternatives to others, I know that we are not alone in finding that they provide answers to problems that do not have conventional remedies.

Of course such alternatives are not infallible, the treatment is not free and we are still grateful for traditional medical and hospital care when necessary. However, it is wonderful that such occasions are now so few and far between. As a result of my experiences I have compiled the information to provide you with the knowledge I wish I had as a new parent.

ACKNOWLEDGEMENTS

I would like to thank all of the following who have given generously of their time to help me write this book: Jane Arnold, Gwen Attwood, Caroline and Eleanor Casterton, Paul and Sally Dean, Sara Drake, Marie Fauré-Anderson, Christine Grabowska, Harriet Griffey, Christine Hall, Anne Mamok, Jane May, Rosamund Parker, Vicki Pitman, Keki Sidwa, Adrian Stoddart, Pat Taylor, David Raitt and Heather Welford. I would particularly like to thank Linda Razzell to whom I am indebted for the information on homeopathy.

PART ONE

THE ALTERNATIVE APPROACH

1.
WHY TRY AN ALTERNATIVE THERAPY?

The first questions to be answered in a book like this are — why should I use alternatives, what can they do for me that my doctor cannot, and are they safe for pregnant mothers and their babies?

The prime reason for choosing to use an alternative approach to any specific health problem is its superior scope. There are many examples of people being cured of ailments for which there is either no equivalent treatment in orthodox medicine, or there is a treatment but it has either not proved effective or is likely to be risky or have side effects. For instance, homeopathic treatment before birth can prevent the baby inheriting family defects. Acupuncture can cure infertility when orthodox treatment has failed. Cranial osteopathy can remedy pyloric stenosis, a potentially dangerous condition in which babies repeatedly vomit their entire feed, by working through the outside of the baby's head as opposed to abdominal operation which is the conventional answer.

Practitioners of alternative medicine aim to enable the body to heal itself. The treatment is of you as a whole and will take into consideration your diet, lifestyle and your feelings about your problem. Although you are only likely to seek help if you have a particular need, their aim is to assist your body to function at its best, so that a pre-conceptual visit can be a sensible step.

Alternative remedies are particularly suited to those who actively want to accept responsibility for the health of themselves and their children. A growing number of people prefer to treat themselves with natural remedies, learning which remedies suit them, and saving antibiotics for life-threatening emergencies. Such people may find the active medical management of modern obstetrics particularly inappropriate and damaging and prefer to assume control of the situation themselves. For them and the midwives who share their belief in the body's ability to give birth without medical intervention are included some of the remedies to ease childbirth which have been used for many years.

Such remedies are not harmless in the sense of being ineffectual, but they are safe to take in the way described. Since the thalidomide disaster, women have rightly been very cautious about taking any drug in pregnancy, and indeed it is usually best to allow your body the opportunity to heal itself. However there are situations, such as with morning sickness, where a remedy is desired. This book offers a range of remedies, with a wider selection for the more common problems. This should make it possible for you to choose a remedy with which you feel happy, which works for you and wherever possible is readily available and inexpensive. However it is important to point out that with long-standing or serious problems it is wise to seek help from a practitioner.

CHOOSING AN ALTERNATIVE PRACTITIONER

Perhaps the best way to find a good alternative therapist is by word of mouth because the majority of therapies would claim to treat most problems and it may be better to choose the person rather than the therapy. However some types of problems are best suited to particular therapies, for instance back and spine problems to osteopathy or chiropractic. Also there may be other factors to bear in mind when making your choice. Some people, for example, are apprehensive about needles and so dislike the idea of acupuncture, while others may be limited by what is available in their area.

If you have not heard of anyone suitable, write to the

respective professional body for a list of their members. Then ring the nearest one, outline your problem and see if you can get a very rough idea of how many treatments you might require. Price can be a drawback, so don't be hesitant about asking about the fees. These can vary widely, usually from £10 upwards, although many therapists say that they would prefer to reduce their fees rather than send someone in urgent need of treatment away. There is often a reduction for children, whom many therapists particularly enjoy treating, because they respond so well and rapidly to treatment. Find out whether they are prepared to prescribe over the phone once they know you. A good practitioner should know his or her limitations and be able to refer you to someone else if they are not able to help.

It can be very refreshing to have an unhurried consultation with a therapist and you should feel that the improvement in your health or solving of your problem makes it worth every penny.

2.
A GUIDE TO ALTERNATIVE THERAPIES

ACUPUNCTURE

This is a complete system of medicine which was developed in China 5,000 years ago. It is based on the theory that the body consists of two opposing parts, Yin and Yang. Yin is deep, cold and female, and Yang is hot, stimulating, male and related to the sun. In good health Yin and Yang are perfectly balanced, but in illness this balance is disturbed.

An acupuncturist will make a diagnosis by taking a full history from you and also by noting your appearance, colour and smell. He or she will then feel your pulses. An acupuncturist can detect as many as 14 separate pulses, and each one tells him a lot about the imbalances within your body. The Chinese believe that the organs of the body are connected by invisible pathways of energy, so that illness in a particular organ may cause pain to be felt in another place along its particular energy pathway or meridian. It is held that illness is caused by obstruction of the energy that should be flowing along these channels and that insertion of the acupuncture needles removes the blockage and allows energy to flow freely again.

The treatment consists of having several very fine needles inserted into different parts of your body for a period of about half an hour. The needles only hurt briefly as they are inserted. Sometimes the acupuncturist may rotate the needles, or send a weak electric current through them. Sometimes dried mugwort or moxa is burned so that heat is transmitted through the needle or directly warms the skin. Once the treatment has been completed, your pulses are checked to ensure that the treatment has been effective. You may feel light-headed or sleepy afterwards. Depending on your need, you may be offered dietary advice and be given further treatments.

The benefits of acupuncture are that no drugs are used and that its scope is far broader than that of Western medicine. Some of its applications are especially suited to pregnancy, for example turning breech babies, or inducing labour so that it starts naturally. Acupuncture is also a superior system of treatment because it frequently proves effective where no orthodox treatment has succeeded, as in some cases of infertility or recurrent miscarriage.

AROMATHERAPY

This is the use of essential plant oils to stimulate, soothe, refresh and heal. The oils are pure distillations from plants and are very concentrated. Some of them have antiseptic properties.

They can be used in various ways, but all of them involve some form of dilution, because they can harm the skin if applied neat. You can add a few drops to your bath, put drops on to a handkerchief, add a little to a bowl of warm water to scent a room, or take a minute amount on a lump of sugar. The oils are often used in massage, when they are diluted in a ratio of one drop of essential oil to $\frac{1}{2}$ teaspoonful (2 ml) of a vegetable oil such as olive or almond. They can also be added to hot water in order to be used as a compress. They are especially suitable for pregnancy and labour.

You can buy the oils from some health shops or order them from G. Baldwin & Co. or Butterbur and Sage Ltd (see page 180). Oils that should be avoided in pregnancy are basil, clove, hyssop, marjoram, myrrh. Oils that should not even be used at home are origanum, sage, savory, thyme, wintergreen.

BACH FLOWER REMEDIES

Discovered by Dr Edward Bach in 1930, there are 38 different remedies. Each one is derived from a flower which has been floated on water in a glass bowl in full sun. The water is preserved with an equal amount of brandy, and bottled. Dr Bach discovered that these remedies had very beneficial effects on negative states of the mind, such as timidity, guilt, lack of confidence, fearfulness, exhaustion.

The remedies are now available from most health shops and you can treat yourself with the aid of Dr Bach's booklet *The Twelve Healers*. You may use more than one remedy at the same time, either putting two drops of each into a glass of water or fruit juice or by making up a solution with 2 tablespoons (30 ml) of water and taking four drops on to the tongue. Add a teaspoonful (5 ml) of brandy or cider vinegar if you want it to keep longer than three weeks. The remedies should be taken at least four times per day.

Rescue Remedy is a combination of five flower remedies — Star of Bethlehem, rock rose, impatiens, cherry plum and clematis. It is extremely useful in cases of mental and physical shock, terror, panic or trauma. Take four drops in water if possible or put it on to the lips and on the pulse points on the wrists and behind the ears.

CRANIAL OSTEOPATHY

A cranial osteopath is a qualified osteopath who specialises in working on your whole body via the fluid and membranes of your brain and spinal cord. They find that by working on the skull they can assess the state of the connective tissue throughout your body and see where old traumas are preventing it from functioning properly. They are then able to remove the impediments which prevent those areas moving in time with the body's internal fluid tide. Correcting them will enable you to function with a good flow of energy and feeling of well-being, and ensure that your body's involuntary mechanisms are working well. Such treatment is especially valuable for pregnant women and babies.

The treatment consists of lying on a couch for 40 minutes while your head is held firmly. You may feel pressure and perhaps subtle changes within it, but it is not painful. You may feel slightly giddy for a few seconds afterwards.

Pregnancy is an especially good time to be treated cranially because the altered hormone levels and changes in the endocrine system makes the connective tissues much softer and more fluid and so better able to alter. The treatment will release any compression in the pelvis so that it is able to stretch fully during the birth. The osteopath will also be working on the sacral nerves which influence the pelvis, cervix and perineum, balancing them so that the cervix dilates smoothly. He or she may also work directly on the pelvis. This treatment is particularly beneficial to women who have had difficulty in giving birth previously.

Cranial treatment can be extremely useful in treating babies too. The pressures that are exerted on their heads during birth are very great, and it can mean that the membranes shear and become twisted as a result. This may be obvious if the head is very moulded or looks asymmetrical. Obviously difficult births are potentially damaging, but even quick and easy births can stress the cranial mechanism. There is a case for suggesting that all babies should receive treatment 14 days after the birth, even those born by elective Caesarean section, because they will have missed the benefits of the rhythmic squeezing and elastic recoil of birth which stimulates pulmonary respiration, and gets the temporal bones moving.

In some cultures grandmothers routinely massage the babies' heads to make them nicely rounded, and well-shaped; people from these cultures have a lower than average incidence of psychological and personality problems.

You may want to take your baby for treatment if it is crying a lot, failing to sleep, hyperactive or if it is frequently sick. Babies do try to help themselves by attempting to expand their palates and open up their cranial mechanisms by means of crying, thumb-sucking and yawning, but they need help. Cranial work can make a miraculous difference to them, often over-night, even to children well past babyhood. It can be especially beneficial for children who are mentally handicapped:

Abigail was born with Down's syndrome and two holes in the heart. She was treated by a cranial osteopath twice a week for four months from birth and then seen weekly for another couple of months. Her holes in the heart closed spontaneously and she is said to be at the top of the intelligence range for a Down's child. Her features still show signs of the syndrome but are not at all marked. Her medical attendants are amazed at how well she has done.

(Details of practitioners can be obtained from the Sutherland Society, see p. 179 for the address.)

HOMEOPATHY

This is a method of enabling the body to heal itself discovered by the German, Samuel Hahnemann, in 1796. He found that giving minute doses of the drugs that caused symptoms identical to those of the disease being treated, actually cured the condition. This established the principle of homeopathy which is 'let like to be cured by like'. The symptoms of illness are seen as the reaction of the body in its attempts to overcome the disease. Homeopathic remedies help the body by strengthening the reaction and allowing the body to heal itself.

For accurate diagnosis and treatment you need to visit a homeopath, who will take a detailed history of your illness and want to know a lot of details about you, what makes you feel better or worse, what kind of temperament you have, your likes and dislikes and so forth, before prescribing a remedy. This will be specifically for you, so that you will get a different remedy to someone else with the same complaint. You can only be sure of getting the correct remedy by visiting a homeopath, although you may be able to consult by phone after the initial visit. For serious or long-standing complaints, a proper consultation is essential. However, a number of the more common remedies are now widely available, and you may want to try them for yourself. If the remedy fails it is because the wrong one has been chosen.

The remedies are available in different strengths; unlike orthodox drugs, the strongest are the most dilute. There are thousands of remedies, prepared largely from plants, although some are made from substances that are regarded as inert, like gold and sand. They are prepared by serial dilution from a mother tincture. This means that one drop of the tincture is diluted with nine or 99 drops of the diluting medium, depending on whether the potency is to be decimal (x) or centesimal (c). The mixture is shaken vigorously, and then one drop from that mixture is taken and diluted again in the same ratio. The first dilution becomes 1c or x, the second 2c or x, etc. The potency generally available is 6c, which is the potency most suitable for self-administration. The c is often omitted so that a remedy might appear as Hepar Sulph 6, for example.

Using the remedies

To use a remedy take one tablet, three times a day for two to three days. In acute conditions take a tablet six times a day, and in very painful conditions such as earache you may need to dose yourself every 15 minutes. When you start to improve, increase the interval between the doses until the improvement is established and then stop. Sometimes the remedy will seem to make the condition worse, in which case stop it altogether. This will probably be followed by a big improvement. Only restart the remedy if the symptoms recur.

In urgent or high energy conditions, such as a fever or

labour, remedies can be given every 5, 10 or 15 minutes as needed. You should generally only take one remedy at a time and avoid other medicines as they may detract from the remedy's efficiency.

The remedies come as tablets or powders, which should be allowed to dissolve under the tongue. They should be taken in a clean mouth, which means you should not have anything to eat or drink for the half hour before or after taking the remedy. Avoid coffee and peppermint while you are using homeopathy, because they may act as antidotes. This may mean you will need to buy one of the toothpastes designed for homeopathy users.

The medicines are sensitive and can easily become contaminated, so you must store them in a cool, dark place away from strong smells. Keep them in their original containers, tip the pills out into the lid so that you do not touch any that you need to put back. If you drop any, do not put the spilled ones back into the bottle. The remedies can also be taken in warm water; this is particularly suitable for acute conditions where doses need to be taken frequently. Crush two tablets and dissolve in warm water.

Babies can be given tablets powdered, either dry or in a little water, or you can put a tablet inside the cheek of a sleeping child.

MEDICAL HERBALISM

Herbs have been used for thousands of years as a gentle and effective way of relieving symptoms and improving general health. They harmonise the body's metabolic processes and correct imbalances within them. Each whole plant is balanced so that within it there are elements which protect the user from the potentially harmful side effects of their active constituents. This is a far safer method of using their healing properties than that employed by modern pharmaceuticals, where drugs are frequently obtained from herbs, but the constituents are isolated and so are without the protective qualities of the rest of the plant.

Herbs do have a physiological effect and so it is best whenever possible to consult a medical herbalist, who will have had an extensive training about the appropriate remedy for your particular needs. He or she will take a detailed history and may give you dietary advice. However herbs have been used safely by ordinary people for many years, and you may want to try some gentle ones yourself. There are some herbs that should be avoided in pregnancy — these are aloe vera, autumn crocus, barberry, broom, juniper, pennyroyal, poke root, parsley, southernwood, tansy, thuja, wormwood, feverfew and sassafras. Goldenseal should not be taken during pregnancy, although it is very useful for stimulating contractions in labour.

There are a number of ways of preparing herbs. You can use them fresh or dried or buy them in a concentrated form such as fluid extracts or tinctures. They can also be obtained as powders which are used to make poultices and pastes or can be put into capsules for swallowing. Herbs are also made up into ointments.

If you are preparing herbs at home it is easiest to make either a decoction or an infusion. An *infusion* or *tea* is made from the aerial parts of a plant — the leaves, stalks or flowers. It is prepared by putting one teaspoonful of the dried herb or three teaspoonsful of the fresh herb into a container, and pouring on a cupful of boiling mineral water. This should then be covered and allowed to stand for 15 minutes without further heating. Strain it and then drink while still warm. A *decoction* is made from the hard parts of plants, such as the roots, rhizomes or stems, which need to be boiled to release their qualities. Cut or crush the herb as much as possible before putting it into a stainless steel or enamel saucepan. Add cold water — 1 pint (600 ml) to 1 oz (25 g) of dried herb, 3 oz (75 g) of fresh — bring it to the boil and simmer it for 15 minutes or more. Allow it to infuse off the heat and then strain it and drink it warm.

Infusions and decoctions should be used within 24 hours. They can be gently reheated to a temperature below boiling, and may be sweetened with honey or made more palatable by the addition of liquorice root.

Fluid extracts and *tinctures* are herbs that have been distilled with water and alcohol respectively. They are very concentrated so that the doses may only be a drop or two in the case of very potent herbs, and is usually between 5–15 drops per dose.

You can obtain a list of practitioners from the National Institute of Medical Herbalists, which has a training clinic in Balham in London where you can be treated by students under supervision for a reduced fee (see p. 179 for the address).

PART TWO

PREGNANCY AND CHILDBIRTH

3.
PLANNING FOR PREGNANCY

Many people conceive unintentionally and many others cannot conceive when they want to, so there are a lot of people to whom the question of timing or preparing for pregnancy does not apply. However there are ways in which you can make sure that the baby you are planning is as healthy as possible, some of which may not be obvious or may require a change of lifestyle. It is well worth considering because taking care of yourself before and during pregnancy does actually make a difference to the health and strength of your baby, and can make the difference between a miserable pregnancy and an enjoyable one.

Firstly, planning. If you are able to think about when you will have a baby, provided conception does not prove a problem, you may want to consider the following:

- When would you want the baby to be born? Winter babies can be fun if you feel that you are going to be quite happy staying in when it is very small, but the amount of wrapping and unwrapping that can be involved can also be a deterrent to getting out and may mean that you end up feeling isolated. Summer babies need less wrapping, but may mean that you are pregnant in the heat which can be enervating.

- Will you lose maternity benefits or your entitlement to maternity rights if you become pregnant now rather than in a few months time? The rules change all the time and you should find out how they apply to you before you become pregnant. Ring your local DHSS office and ask for the current leaflets on maternity benefits.

- If you already have children at school or nursery, will you be in the early months of the pregnancy in the holidays when you are likely to feel your most tired; will the baby be due during the holidays and would this be an advantage or not?

- March conceptions can be Christmas babies — it is worth thinking about the baby's birthday and subsequent parties, usually much easier if there is a chance that they can be held outside.

- If you plan to move house or have building work done while pregnant — a surprising number of people do — can you avoid it happening in the early or late months of the pregnancy (most people can't)?

PRE-CONCEPTUAL CARE

A list of health considerations for a planned pregnancy include:

- Stop taking the contraceptive pill at least three months before trying to get pregnant. Some, as yet unsubstantiated studies, suggest there is a higher risk of defects, such as cleft palate, in babies conceived immediately after stopping the pill.

- Pay attention to your daily food intake, cutting out or down on refined foods, such as biscuits, cakes, sweets, high-fat foods like chips, and foods that contain large amounts of sugar, additives and artificial colourings. Eat fresh rather than manufactured goods, concentrating on meat, fish, cheese, wholegrains, pulses, fruit and vegetables. If you are a vegetarian make sure that you are taking a vitamin B12 supplement, and maybe a multivitamin. Also avoid eating raw or undercooked meats and do not drink unpasteurised milk or soft cheeses.

- Cut out, or at least down, on alcohol and smoking. Smoking affects the baby directly giving rise to babies of lower birth weight who may be born prematurely, suffer the consequences of pregnancy complications, and be susceptible to respiratory infections after birth. Alcohol should be avoided, especially around the time of conception, and during pregnancy, particularly in the first three months. Alcohol addiction in a woman who is pregnant can lead to her baby being born with fetal alcohol syndrome where the baby has distinctive facial features and is likely to be mentally retarded. The safe limit for alcohol is not known and is likely to vary between individuals, so that it is simplest to avoid it altogether if possible or at least for the first three months of pregnancy. Acupuncture can help treat addictions.

- Get fit — by swimming, cycling or some other type of all-round exercise. Pregnancy makes considerable demands on the body and labour itself can take a significant physical toll. Both can be easier if you start off in good physical shape.

- Try to get any long-standing problems cleared up; these might include systemic candida (see p. 78), allergies, and so on. If you think there may be any type of inherited defect that could be passed on to your children, it would be wise to seek some genetic counselling. Some of these types of problems can be treated homeopathically.

- Stop any drugs that are not essential. You may need to discuss this with your GP or consultant, or seek advice from a pre-conception clinic. It may also be worth consulting an alternative practitioner if you have a problem for which you need to take drugs in pregnancy. There is always the chance that you can be treated so effectively that you no longer require the drugs. Cut out drugs such as aspirin too.

- Try to cut out tea and coffee, and other caffeine-containing substances, such as chocolate and cola, which may be harmful to the foetus.

- Check your rubella status by having a blood test done to see whether you are immune to German measles. If you are not then have the immunisation, but be sure to allow three months between having the immunisation and trying to conceive.

- Avoid environmental hazards as far as possible; these include things that are intended to kill such as woodworm killer, insecticides, weedkiller. Also watch out for lead fumes from stripping old paint, hair spray and dyes, mercury amalgam at the dentist, cooking with aluminium, medication if it can be avoided, including treatment for threadworms and nits, radiation from X rays and debatably VDUs. A general proviso would be to avoid anything that makes you feel ill or which you intuitively feel will not be good for your baby. The London Hazards Centre will advise you about individual substances that concern you (see p. 183 for address), and Foresight, an organisation for pre-conceptual care, can organise hair analysis which may reveal toxic metal overload (address on p. 182).

Obviously, there are occasions where you are unable to avoid some of these hazards and clearly instinct does not work for everyone, particularly in those whose addictions overwhelm their intuition. However most women find that even in very early pregnancy they find they go off things that are potentially damaging. Alcohol, cigarettes and coffee are frequently felt to be nauseating and one should obey these instincts. Women sometimes find other things that are less obviously harmful intolerable, too, such as fatty and spicy foods. Equally it can be surprising to find yourself craving foods that you normally dislike. Providing they are not obviously damaging, you can indulge these instincts.

The first 13–14 weeks of pregnancy are those in which the baby's organs and limbs are being formed and these are the weeks in which it is most important to avoid taking anything which could cause the baby to be malformed. The time around conception is thought to be especially important. As it is not until your period is due that you can confirm a pregnancy, this means being careful from *before* ovulation onwards.

4.
PROBLEMS WITH CONCEIVING

As many as one in six couples have problems with fertility, although a problem is usually recognised as existing only when conception has not occurred after at least a year of trying. The causes range from the mechanical, such as scar tissue as a consequence of pelvic disease, or a complete absence of sperm, through to the unexplained infertility where tests show that everything is functioning well and yet there is no pregnancy.

Some problems can only be treated by surgery. For instance, if both of the hairsbreadth Fallopian tubes are blocked, it is unlikely that alternative treatments will help. However alternative treatments *do* treat infertility successfully in many cases where orthodox treatment has failed.

Any couple failing to become pregnant would first be advised to look at their diet (see p. 18) and lifestyle and see if there is room for improvement. Although it is quite possible to become pregnant on a very limited diet and whilst under great stress, these conditions can cause infertility in some individuals. It is also an area which tends to be ignored by infertility clinics, so that you could be attending the clinic for months whilst living on coffee and lettuce leaves, your stress level pushed ever higher by all the tensions and anguish commonly felt by those seeking treatment. An inadequate diet, and even a good one, may not be providing some of the trace elements which can be essential for conception. Even those eating well may, for some reason of individual metabolism, be deficient in some elements.

Supplements suggested by Drs Stephen Davies and

Alan Stewart in their comprehensive book *Nutritional Medicine* are as follows:

FOR WOMEN

Follow dietary advice on p. 18. Take a broad spectrum multivitamin and mineral supplement and vitamin E, 200–400 IUs daily (though Susun Weed suggests that 500–1500 IUs taken daily can prevent birth defects in children of couples who have defective children).

FOR MEN

Daily doses of:
Multivitamin and mineral supplement
Elemental zinc, 50 mg
Vitamin C, 200–500 mg
Lysine, 500 mg
Arginine, 1.5–2 g
Free-form amino acids, 500 mg twice daily
Vitamin E, 200–400 IUs (see above).

Conventional treatment starts by checking that ovulation is taking place, so that if you are considering seeing your doctor because of fertility problems it is a good idea to have already made basal body temperature (BBT) charts (see p. 29 for details of how to go about doing this). A sperm count can be run fairly readily and this will show whether there are adequate numbers of sperm, whether they are healthy and if they are able to move freely. If ovulation is not occurring even though you may be having periods, it can be boosted with drugs. Excessive exercise can prevent ovulation.

A low sperm count is less easily treated, although lowering the temperature of the testicles by bathing them in cool water, wearing boxer shorts and losing weight if over-weight, can help because the testes need to be cool to function properly.

If ovulation is taking place and the sperm count is adequate the next step is likely to be laparoscopy, the internal examination of the woman's pelvic cavity by means of a fibre-optic telescope inserted through a small incision made just below the navel. This is done under general anaesthetic. With the help of the laparoscope, the surgeon can see if there are adhesions caused by pelvic infection or a condition, endometriosis, caused by tissue from the lining of the uterus growing outside it, yet bleeding monthly and forming cysts. (See *Understanding Endometriosis*, Caroline Hawkridge, Optima). Adhesions can mean that the Fallopian tubes are not free to move to scoop up the egg, or that their ends are stuck together or that they are affected in some way which prevents fertilisation taking place. Blocked tubes can be tested for by means of filling the uterus with dye and examining its progress up the tubes on an X-ray. An alternative test is to blow air through them.

One or more of these tests may reveal a problem which can only be dealt with by surgery, or complex techniques such as in-vitro fertilisation. However the largest group of infertile couples are those for whom there is no evident barrier to conception and it is these for whom the following alternative treatments may result in pregnancy.

ALTERNATIVE TREATMENTS FOR INFERTILITY

Acupuncture
There have been some remarkable successes with acupuncture to treat both male and female infertility. An acupuncturist would treat you individually and might advise you about diet. Acupuncture can also help women who conceive easily but miscarry repeatedly.

Lindsay sought the help of an acupuncturist because she had glandular fever and her low blood pressure was resulting in her fainting frequently. She had been trying to get pregnant for 18 months but with no success. The blood pressure problem was alleviated by the first treatment, and subsequently her periods were regularised and her ovarian cysts dispersed. She had acupuncture monthly at ovulation to strengthen her body's reactions, and to make her fit to maintain a pregnancy. Her husband had acupuncture to improve a low sperm count, and within two months she was pregnant. She had treatment to maintain her strength, and the baby was treated in utero at 14 and 26 weeks to ensure that it had a good digestion, was strong and had plenty of hair. She took zinc throughout and gave birth to a boy without difficulty. She also found that using lavender and Neroli essential oils in a base prevented stretch marks.

Homeopathy
Homeopathy can work well in cases of infertility. Treatment must be from a homeopath.

Medical herbalism
It would be best to consult a practitioner for an individual diagnosis, although there are herbs that you can try. For women there are red clover flowers — combine 1 oz (25 g) of flowers with a teaspoon (5 ml) of peppermint and infuse with 2 pints (1.2 litres) of water, drink it freely throughout the day. Nettle tea and raspberry leaf tea should also be taken daily, at least a cupful each day. False unicorn root is good for correcting hormonal imbalances and can be taken as a tincture 5–15 drops daily. The berries of the chaste tree, *Vitex Agnus castus*, have an unrivalled reputation for their ability to affect the pituitary gland and normalise oestrogen and progesterone output. It can be taken as tablets, two three times a day. For pelvic infection try false unicorn root (*Helonias*) and blue cohosh. For ovarian dysfunction try *Agnus castus* + *Helonias*.

Men should try oats and sarsaparilla.

Cranial osteopathy
By working through the bones of your head, a cranial osteopath can affect the action of the pea-sized pituitary gland which governs the output of hormones. This can be particularly useful for women whose periods are irregular or who are not ovulating.

Some cranial osteopaths work directly on the organs through the abdomen, which can free adhesions and get the uterus working normally.

Sharon had not become pregnant although she and her husband had been trying for two years. She had cranial treatment to improve the function of her pituitary gland and get her hormones functioning better, and work on her pelvis to improve the drainage from the uterus and improve the blood supply to the ovaries. Within two months she was pregnant and went on to have a healthy boy. Three years later she had not managed to conceive again and further treatment eventually resulted in her having a daughter. She subsequently became pregnant without treatment.

Hypnotherapy

It can be hard to accept that infertility can be affected by the mind and that for some unconscious reason you are not allowing pregnancy to take place, even harder perhaps that your subconscious can maintain this hold even when you are asleep. However everyone knows of at least one person who has been unable to conceive and yet become pregnant once they adopt a baby, or is told there is nothing more that can be done medically and then finds that they have conceived without any assistance at all.

Hypnotherapy can, on occasion, deal with the matters that trouble the subconscious of both men and women so that the brakes which prevent conception are removed. Contact the British Hypnotherapy Association for details (see p. 178).

5.
CONCEPTION

It might seem as though conception is the easy part —
after all, you have probably been practising for years.
However, having made the decision to have a baby, you will
be keen to start it straightaway and it is useful to know
when to try. There is in each month, in fact, only a
surprisingly short time for which you are fertile. This
information becomes useful later to avoid pregnancy.

THE FERTILITY CYCLE

Ovulation, the release of an egg from the ovary, ripe for
fertilisation, takes place roughly 14 days before a period
starts. This means it is mid-way through a 28-day cycle,
but could be a week later, ie 21 days after the start of a
period, for someone with a 35-day cycle. If you have
regular cycles, timing conception should be relatively easy,
but if you cannot be certain when your next period is due,
there are other ways of working out when ovulation is
taking place.

Conception takes place when a sperm meets and
fertilises an egg or ovum, after it has been released from
the ovary where it has been ripening. The egg develops in
a follicle on the ovary; boosted by hormones, the follicle
eventually bursts and discharges the egg (occasionally two)
into the pelvic cavity where it is scooped up by the mobile
fringe of one of the Fallopian tubes, and is wafted down
the tube towards the uterus. Although sperm can survive
for three to five days, the egg only lives for 12–24 hours, so
that for fertilisation to take place, intercourse should
either have occurred within the two or three days prior to
ovulation or within the few hours after it. In the
circumstances it seems astonishing that over-population
could ever be a problem.

CHARTING OVULATION

The ways in which you can work out when you ovulate are by taking your temperature daily, being aware of the changes in the mucus from the cervix, and possibly by individual body signs. There are also a couple of commercial tests available.

Even if you do not know when you ovulate you may be aware that the type of mucus discharge from your vagina changes in quality and quantity throughout the month. With practice you can become familiar with the different types and recognise the kind that indicates you are about to ovulate. It may be easiest to start by directly feeling your cervix every day. The best way to do this is by washing your hands, leaving them wet and then squatting or sitting on the loo. Insert one or two fingers into your vagina and push them up as far as they will go. The cervix at the top of your vagina will feel like a firm smooth knob, with a little indentation in the middle which is the os or opening. The uterus is attached in the pelvis by ligaments so that it is slightly mobile and its position in relation to the vagina alters during the month. At the start of the cycle it is low, rising by 2–3 cm at ovulation to its highest point, when it is hardest to reach with your fingers, and then becoming low in the vagina again as your period approaches. At ovulation the os changes from being tightly closed to gaping slightly, and the vagina becomes softer and more accommodating.

The most striking difference, however, is in the amount and texture of the mucus coming from the cervix during the course of the menstrual cycle. Mucus which follows a period is fairly scanty, sticky, dry, opaque and paste-like. As the time of ovulation approaches the mucus becomes much wetter and more slippery. It also clears, becomes more profuse, and stretchy so that you can string it between two fingers — it has a consistency not unlike egg white at this time. There may be sufficient quantities of mucus to make your underpants feel wet. This change in mucus occurs at ovulation in order to enable the sperm to swim rapidly through it and up the cervical canal. In ideal conditions they can reach the Fallopian tubes in 5 minutes.

Once ovulation has taken place, indicated by a peak day with the maximum mucus loss, the cervix and mucus return quite rapidly to their pre-ovulatory state, when the cervix is low and hard, the os is closed and the mucus is cloudier, stickier and less plentiful. If you are using your fertility awareness as a method of contraception you should be safe following the third day after the peak day.

You can also tell when you are ovulating by a method known as basal body temperature (BBT) charting. This involves taking your temperature daily, either first thing in the morning before you get up or at another set time, provided in both instances that you have nothing to eat or drink for an hour beforehand. Buy a fertility thermometer from a chemist, and using graph paper plot a chart with the days of the month along one axis and the possible range of temperatures along the other. It may be between 36.0°C and 37.0°C, but depends on individual variation. Take your temperature and then plot the result on the graph (this can be done later in the day if more convenient). At the end of your cycle, join the dots and you should have a chart with consistently lower readings in the first half of the cycle than in the second. In between the levels there should be a slight drop followed within a day or two by a noticeable rise of 0.2°C–0.5°C. This indicates that ovulation has taken place. Charts are not always easy to interpret and can be affected by illness, so they are best used in conjunction with the other signs.

Other ways of anticipating ovulation include various body changes. These might be insomnia, tiredness, increased sex drive, fullness and tenderness of the breasts, vaginal odour, spots, greasiness of hair. You might also feel cramp-like pains on the right or left side of the body depending on which ovary has released the egg, vulval pressure, pains in the legs or nettle-rash or other symptoms specific to you. Careful observation of your cycle will mean that you become well aware of your fertility and so able to pick the right time to attempt conception.

The commercial tests available from the chemist can be used to detect the surge in luteinising hormone which means that ovulation is going to take place in the next 12–24 hours. They are expensive, but claim accuracy of prediction of around 66 per cent for the first month of testing increasing to 85 per cent if used for longer. They can prove if you are failing to ovulate at all.

TIMING SEXUAL INTERCOURSE

In order to give yourself the best opportunity of becoming pregnant, have sex every other day from the day your cervical mucus starts to become wet, until you are sure you have ovulated. You need only have sex once at ovulation — sex more frequently than every 48 hours can deplete the level of sperm. Make love in the conventional position, with a pillow under your bottom. Your partner should wait until his penis is limp before withdrawing and your should stay on your back for half an hour. MAKE A NOTE OF THE DATE IN YOUR DIARY.

CHOOSING THE SEX OF YOUR CHILD

Having sex around the time of ovulation should mean you get pregnant, but you may particularly want a boy or girl. You can alter the odds so that you get a 80–85 per cent chance of having a baby of the sex you want. In order to do this you need to be as sure as possible of your time of ovulation, and plan sex carefully around that time.

For a boy
Abstain from sex for at least four days before ovulation; then have sex as close as possible to the moment of ovulation. Before intercourse, give yourself a vaginal douche with water with sodium bicarbonate dissolved in it, in a dilution of 1 tablespoonful (15 ml) to a pint (600 ml) of water. If you do not have a douche bag, fill a well-rinsed

soft plastic detergent bottle with the water, insert the nozzle and squeeze the sides until the fluid floods your vagina. This produces the alkaline conditions which favour male (Y) sperm. Alkaline mucus is also produced by orgasm and this together with full penetration at ejaculation also helps.

For a girl
Deliberately conceiving a girl is less easy as it requires anticipating the time of ovulation and having sex two or three days beforehand. You must then abstain until three days after ovulation. The douche for a girl is 1 tablespoon (15 ml) of white vinegar to a pint (600 ml) of water. The theory is that female sperm outlive male ones and so they are the ones still in the Fallopian tubes when the egg is released. The X sperm travel most easily in acid conditions.

THE FIRST SYMPTOMS OF PREGNANCY

Most people who have been pregnant once have a pretty good idea when they have conceived on subsequent occasions. The first time it is less easy to be certain and it is in the gap between conception and the time when a period would be due that one wants to know, now that you can get a result from a home pregnancy test the day that you are due.

The fertilised egg travels down the Fallopian tube, taking about five to seven days to reach the uterus. Once there the multiplying cells burrow into the endometrium, the lining of the uterus. This implantation site is the one where the placenta will develop. Some women actually feel implantation as strong contractions lasting several hours. Occasionally there is a very slight blood loss.

From this time onward you may feel some of the symptoms of early pregnancy. Your breasts may feel tender or throb or tingle. They may swell and itch or you might feel shooting pains in them. You may also be much thirstier and hungrier than usual, and as a result you may need to go to the toilet more frequently. You might feel dizzy or unusually warm.

You will probably feel devastatingly tired, and be ready to go to bed in the early evening, if not before. Often your digestion is completely upset and you may have feelings of nausea or actually be sick. Some food and drink may completely lose its appeal, typically fatty food, coffee, alcohol, and you may have cravings for some foods you don't normally like. Your sense of smell can be upset too, some smells can become nauseating and you can be haunted by unpleasant smells which no-one else can smell. You may also have a metallic taste in your mouth.

If you have all these symptoms you are almost certainly pregnant, but there are two other ways of telling. One is by means of your cervix. If you are pregnant your cervix remains high and grows increasingly soft instead of becoming lower and hard as it usually does before a period. At the same time your vagina gradually changes colour from its usual pink to a dusky purple-blue. The second way is if you have been taking your temperature. You are likely to be pregnant if your temperature stays high at the end of your cycle and does not drop just before the period is due, as it would normally. A temperature above 37.2°C suggests pregnancy.

6.
PREPARING YOURSELF FOR PREGNANCY AND BIRTH

DIET

Diet is of vital importance to the pregnant and lactating woman and to her growing baby. The baby is totally dependent on its mother for all its nutrients and it seems obvious that it should only be getting the best. Moreover well-nourished women tend to do much better in labour and their babies are born in better condition and are more healthy overall. There are two situations when it is easy to overlook this wisdom. The first is if you suffer from morning sickness when it can be difficult to keep anything at all down and almost any healthy food can seem quite repulsive. The other is when you have been pregnant for some months, it seems most unlikely that you will ever be anything else and therefore no point in being careful about what you eat.

Ideally you will be eating well before your conceive, but if not you should take time to work out a good diet once you are pregnant and able to tolerate a wide range of foods. It is important to avoid the Mars bar and cup of coffee syndrome even when very rushed. If this is your first baby it can be difficult to modify your behaviour for its benefit because it is much harder to visualise it and be protective towards it. Your needs are all too obvious whereas the baby's have to be guessed at. A good diet will help you feel better too though and more able to cope with the demands pregnancy makes of your system.

Try to make sure that you eat at least three times a day. As you grow and there is less room in your stomach, it can be better to eat six small meals daily. Some general rules would include the following:

- Avoid refined carbohydrates, making sure that most of your calories come from whole grains, potatoes, beans and pulses.

- Eat plenty of fresh fruit and vegetables, at least some of them raw.

- Eat 60–80 g of protein daily. This can be chosen from meat, fish, eggs, milk and dairy products.

- Eat dried fruit and nuts for snacks.

- Drink plenty of spring water.

- Avoid tea and coffee.

Nutritional supplementation

Nutritional supplementation in pregnancy is a controversial issue. You may feel that you are eating well and that all nutrients are best obtained from food and that taking vitamins and minerals is potentially risky. On the other hand, you could feel that the baby's needs put a strain on your resources which for various reasons such as poor health, poor diet, stress or exhaustion are not at their best, and that as a result you want to provide the best for both of you by taking extra supplements. Some are suggested in the following pages.

Vitamin supplements taken prior to conception and in pregnancy have been shown to reduce the numbers of babies born with spina bifida to mothers who have previously had affected babies and whose subsequent children were at increased risk of being born with the condition.

Zinc deficiency seems to be a common finding in non-pregnant women and it is one of the things, together with folic acid, vitamin B, vitamin C, calcium and magnesium, for which there is a 30–100 per cent increase in need in pregnancy. Your diet does have to be good to meet these requirements.

If you wish to take supplements, a recommended regime would be:

1 multivitamin
1 vitamin B complex
1 g vitamin C
3 Dolomite tablets (calcium and magnesium)
15 mg zinc

Vegans and vegetarians are advised to make sure they include a 3–4 micrograms of vitamin B12 daily in their diets, even if they do not take the other supplements.

One note of warning here, no pregnant woman should take more than 7,500 to 10,000 IUs of vitamin A per day as this can cause malformations.

Natural ways of obtaining vitamins and minerals

The following list shows which vitamins and minerals can be found in which foods and plants.

VITAMIN A — green, yellow or orange vegetables, margarine, orange and yellow fruits, alfalfa, watercress, parsley, nettles, raspberry leaf.
VITAMIN B COMPLEX — whole grains, pork, beef, liver, beans, cereals, brown rice, milk, dairy produce, eggs, bananas, avocados, nuts, seeds.
VITAMIN B6 — meat, fish, egg yolk, whole grains, bananas, avocados, seeds, nuts.
VITAMIN B12 — liver, offal, meat, fish, dairy produce, eggs, brewer's yeast, alfalfa, comfrey, miso, and seaweed.
VITAMIN C — most fruits, green vegetables, liver, kidney, potatoes, elderberries, rosehips.
FOLIC ACID — liver, kidney, green vegetables, eggs, wholegrain cereals.
VITAMIN D — fatty fish, cod liver oil, eggs, milk, butter, margarine, cheese, alfalfa, nettles, sunshine.

VITAMIN E — vegetable oils, nuts, seeds, soya, lettuce, eggs, watercress, alfalfa, rosehips, raspberry leaf, dandelion, seaweed.

VITAMIN K — turnips, greens, broccoli, cabbage, lettuce, liver, green tea, cereals, alfalfa, nettles, kelp.

CALCIUM — milk, cheese, broccoli, green leafy vegetables, nuts, seeds, peas, beans, lentils, alfalfa, red clover, raspberry leaf, comfrey, nettles, parsley, watercress.

PHOSPHORUS — milk and dairy produce, nuts, whole grains, cereals, poultry, eggs, meat and fish, caraway seeds, parsley, watercress, nettles, chickweed, alfalfa, liquorice, marigold petals, raspberry leaf.

POTASSIUM — fresh fruits, vegetables, whole grains, chamomile, comfrey, dandelion, parsley.

MAGNESIUM — nuts, winkles, shrimps, soya, whole grains, green leafy vegetables, tap water in hard water areas, watercress, alfalfa, parsley, carrot tops.

IRON — liver, kidney, heart, egg yolk, peas, beans, cocoa, molasses, shellfish, parsley, nettles, dandelion, alfalfa, yellow dock.

SILICON — spinach, horsetail, dandelion, nettles, leeks.

MANGANESE — leafy green vegetables, whole grains, spinach, alfalfa, parsley, watercress.

FLUORINE — spinach, watercress, garlic.

CHROMIUM — brewer's yeast, whole grains, liver, cheese, molasses.

COPPER — oysters, kidney, liver, dried peas and beans, nuts, spinach, cabbage, watercress, alfalfa, parsley, kale, nettles, chickweed.

SODIUM — salt, milk, cheese.

SELENIUM — eggs, fish, whole grains, brown rice, meat, poultry, nuts.

SULPHUR — cabbage family vegetables, nettles, plantain, coltsfoot, garlic.

IODINE — shrimps, fish, beef liver, pineapple, eggs, peanuts, wholewheat bread, raisins, watercress, parsley, sarsaparilla, seaweeds.

ZINC — oysters, lamb chops, steak, pecan nuts, split

peas, brazil nuts, beef liver, non-fat dried milk, egg yolk, whole wheat, rye, oats, peanuts, watercress.

AMINO ACIDS (INCLUDING LYSINE AND ARGININE) — found in all first-class protein such as meat, fish, eggs and dairy products.

Supplements to prepare for labour
Some of the remedies designed to ease labour have to be taken during pregnancy. Raspberry leaf tea or tablets, possibly combined with mitchella or squaw vine is one such remedy. The tea can be taken once a day throughout pregnancy or three times a day for the last three months. It is rich in iron and vitamin C and is an aid to digestion. It tones the uterus and helps to prevent haemorrhage.

There is also a Pre-Natal Formula sold by Self-Heal Herbs, which combines squaw vine, holy thistle, black cohosh, pennyroyal, false unicorn, raspberry leaves and lobelia. It is taken for the last six weeks and is good for women who have had difficult births previously, or who are not in good health.

The homeopathic equivalent is Caullophyllum, and this has been recommended as a prophylactic against a difficult labour. However it is now felt that, as with any homeopathic remedy, it can be counter-productive to take it routinely or when there is no indicated need. It can in fact cause the symptoms that you are trying to avoid, in this case slow inefficient contractions, and can slow or stop labour and may result in bleeding. It does have a place if you are under threat of induction, or if the waters have gone and contractions have not started. If it fails to start labour under these circumstances consult a homeopath.

EXERCISE

Most women are keen to make giving birth as easy as possible, and there are a number of ways of preparing for the birth that should ensure that you are fit for the event.

Exercise is one of the ways of getting in training. You can book into yoga classes specifically for pregnancy at the birth centres around the country, the National Childbirth Trust (NCT) incorporate exercise in their ante-natal classes and there are many other types of pregnancy exercise classes available. If you cannot reach a class, you can follow your own exercise routine at home. A good programme is set out in *New Life* by Janet and Arthur Balaskas, for example.

Swimming and cycling are particularly helpful forms of exercise. Swimming uses every muscle in your body and the water supports your weight, something that becomes increasingly welcome as pregnancy progresses. Cycling too takes your weight while you get fitter and it can also help to widen your pelvic outlet.

Two exercises that are important and which should be practised daily are the *pelvic floor exercise* and *squatting*. You should be able to spend as long as 15 minutes in an unsupported squat by the end of pregnancy, although for various reasons not everyone manages this. When you first start, you may find that you need the support of a wall and need to put a couple of books under your heels. However if you practise squatting every day you will eventually be able to squat unsupported with your heels flat on the floor, your back straight and your knees apart. If you clasp your hands together under your chin you can use your elbows to separate your knees.

The pelvic floor exercise is useful for toning up the muscles around your perineum and it teaches control of those muscles so that you are able to relax them consciously at the moment of crowning. It is especially important to do the pelvic floor exercise after the birth to help tone up the pelvic muscles which will have been stretched. Doing the exercise daily should reduce the risk of uterine prolapse in later life.

To do the exercise first try and identify the muscles by trying to stop yourself in mid-flow of urine. These are the muscles you need to exercise. Practise drawing them up slowly, holding them at their tightest for several seconds, and then slowly letting go. Try doing five at a time, several times a day.

Your capacity for exercise decreases as you get closer to the birth, but it is important to maintain your activity because labour is usually a time that uses up a lot of strength and energy and the fitter you are the easier it is to cope.

PERINEAL MASSAGE

Massaging your perineum from about 30 weeks of pregnancy can help to make it more supple and stretchy, so that is better able to slide over the baby's head, rather than tearing, during the birth. Massage can also help to soften previous episiotomy scars.

The best time to start the massage is after a warm bath. Using an oil such as comfrey, almond, olive, vitamin E, wheatgerm or calendula ointment, lubricate your fingers. Then very gently insert two fingers into your vagina and gradually increase the space between them so that the skin becomes stretched, a bit like pulling out the corners of your mouth. You will find that as time goes by you will be able to accommodate more of your fingers. Hook your thumb into your vagina and pull the perineum outward, massaging the skin with the oil in a U-shape while concentrating on any area of tenderness or previous scar. You will find that the whole area softens as you get closer to delivery, but massaging daily can make a real difference to your perineum.

ANTE-NATAL CLASSES

Ante-natal classes may provide an opportunity for you to discuss particular anxieties and share the experience of becoming parents with others at a similar stage. As in all self-help groups, the members will provide a special understanding which can only be obtained from those who are feeling just the way you are at present. You can join classes organised by your hospital, clinic, the National

Childbirth Trust, or birth centre (see pp. 181–85 addresses).

BIRTH ATTENDANTS

One way of making your birth easier is to have someone with you, as well or instead of the baby's father. This might be someone who has had children herself, who will know intuitively how you are feeling and how you can be helped and who also feels the excitement and privilege of being at a birth. Although it is not customary in this country at present, evidence from a large study in America shows that the presence of 'doulas' — lay birth companions — has a very positive effect in terms of outcome and duration of labour. It can be enormously helpful to have a sympathetic person with you, someone who has been through it herself, who will provide support and comfort, even though you have a partner and midwife with you. If you would like someone with you, but do not know anyone to ask, you could try asking your ante-natal teacher — many would be thrilled to be asked. If you are planning a hospital birth, make sure well in advance that you will be able to have the people of your choice with you. Some hospitals have policies limiting you to one partner only, but this is subject to negotiation.

REBIRTHING

This is one way of preparing yourself for childbirth. It is a simple breathing technique that works on the principle that there is a direct connection between physical and mental well-being and that breathing is the key element in liberating the body from tension, fear and pain. It can help you to become more in touch with your feelings and allows you to recognise and release hurtful memories. (See p. 179 for address of the Rebirth Society.)

7.
AN A–Z OF POSSIBLE PROBLEMS AND THEIR REMEDIES

ANAEMIA

A sample of your blood will be taken several times during your pregnancy to test, among other things, for the haemoglobin level. Haemoglobin (Hb) is a measure of the quantity and quality of the red oxygen-carrying cells in your body. The scale is from 14.7 g downwards and you are considered anaemic if your Hb is 11 g or lower. Anaemia is more likely to occur in the last three months or so of pregnancy when the baby's need for iron is greatest. Anaemia can make you feel very tired and deplete your reserves so that blood loss at delivery could be serious, which is why women are often given iron and folic acid supplements routinely. However the value of routine supplementation is being questioned, partly because only 7 per cent of pregnant women suffer from anaemia anyway, and partly because high levels of iron are thought to predispose towards post-partum haemorrhage, and may make the red cells bigger so that they are unable to cross the placenta. Iron supplements can also give you jet black stools, cause constipation and piles and make some women feel sick.

The best way to avoid the need for iron tablets is to make sure that you include plenty of iron-rich foods in your diet. Good sources of iron include lean meat, especially liver and kidney, wheatgerm, watercress, dried fruit, celeriac, butter beans, kidney beans, dark green vegetables, cream, cottage cheese and cocoa.

If you know you are anaemic, you could try taking Floradix in liquid or tablet form; this is a herbal preparation which is rich in iron. Iron is better assimilated by the body if it is taken along with vitamin C. Certain foods, such as bran, tea and coffee, can actually inhibit the body's ability to absorb iron from food, so should be avoided if possible. Tea drunk at meal times seem to be the most harmful.

It is quite possible that you may not need any supplementation if you are eating a properly balanced diet. Moreover, you may be clinically anaemic and yet feel fine. It is thought by some people that some degree of anaemia is normal because of the great increase in blood volume in pregnancy. The haemoglobin returns to normal after delivery when a lot of excess fluid is shed.

If you are tired but not anaemic you may be helped by taking 1–3 g of oil of evening primrose.

Acupuncture
You can be treated successfully by acupuncture so it would be worth seeking specialist advice.

Homeopathic remedies
Similarly with homeopathic remedies, it is best to consult a homeopath for an individual diagnosis, although Ferrum or Ferrum Magneticum 9 c potency helps anaemia in many women.

BACKACHE (see also Sacro-iliac joint pain)

Backache can seem an inevitable part of pregnancy. It occurs partly as a consequence of the softening effect the hormone relaxin has on your ligaments, in preparation for giving birth, and partly as a result of carrying the weight of the growing baby at the front of your body. This additional weight tends to make you thrust your shoulders back and your stomach forward in order to maintain your balance, and this invariably puts a strain on your spine.

It is easier to take steps to prevent backache than it is to cure it once it has started. You can help yourself by maintaining the strength of your back through exercising. Such exercises are best started before pregnancy, but they will help even if you are already suffering from backache. Swimming is the best form of exercise, and yoga is very helpful too.

The other method of prevention is by paying careful attention to your posture. Try to think about balancing the baby in your pelvis like an egg in an egg cup. Do this by making the angle of your pelvis less by flattening the curve of your back and bending your knees slightly when standing. It is not always easy to remember to do this, but you can get into the habit of it if you practise for a while. It is particularly important to adopt this posture if you are standing for any length of time.

Shoes with even a slight heel can put an extra strain on your back, so it is best to wear flat-heeled shoes throughout pregnancy. It will also help to sit upright on a hard chair rather than slouching on a sofa, and to sleep on a reasonably hard mattress. Put boards underneath the mattress of your bed if it is too soft.

Some women are helped by wearing a maternity girdle available in specialist corsetry shops or department stores. It may also help to take a calcium supplement — 6 tablets of Dolomite daily. Remember that vomiting while bending over a loo or a basin can damage your spine. Problems in your dorsal spine can irritate the vagus nerve leading to the stomach and lead to further vomiting, resulting in a vicious circle of illness.

Homeopathic remedies
If your spine or sacrum or hips feel weak and you feel worse for stooping and walking, take Aesculus. If you feel exhausted and have a burning in the spine and the small of your back feels weak, it is worse in cold weather and on

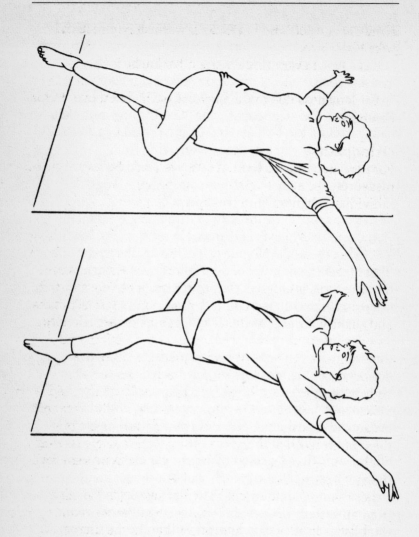

The following hip rotation exercise helps relieve backache. Lie flat on your back and stretch your arms out to the side. Keep one leg straight and hook the foot of the other under your calf. Keeping your shoulders on the ground, twist your hips so that the knee of the bent leg touches the ground as nearly as possible. Hold for a few seconds and then repeat the exercise using the alternate leg. Also try crawling on all fours, keeping your spine straight and your pelvis tucked under you. Exercises taught at yoga or ante-natal exercise classes will help too.

lying on your left and better with warmth and motion, take Kali Carb.

Take Arica every three hours if backache is due to over-exertion.

For lameness due to the pressure of the baby take Bellis Perennis.

Osteopathy
For persistent backache that is not relieved by any of these measures, see an osteopath or chiropractor for an individual diagnosis and treatment.

BLEEDING IN PREGNANCY

Slight bleeding in pregnancy does not necessarily mean that the fetus is at risk. Although it is not common it does occur in around 10 per cent of pregnancies up to 28 weeks and slightly fewer after that time. It may be experienced as a slight loss at the time of the expected period, and sometimes at 14 weeks when the placenta takes over hormone production from the corpus luteum (a yellow body which grows on the ovary in place of the ruptured follicle and which sustains the pregnancy until this point). It can also be caused by cervical polyps and erosions — these often bleed after intercourse which is disconcerting but has no effect on the pregnancy. They can be seen with the aid of a speculum.

Less common, but potentially dangerous, is bleeding from an ectopic pregnancy. This is when the pregnancy establishes itself somewhere other than in the uterus, generally in one of the Fallopian tubes. Bleeding starts sometime between 6–12 weeks and it may be accompanied by one-sided abdominal pain. The growing embryo eventually distends the tube until it ruptures, causing pain, shock and bleeding both internally and from the vagina. Surgery is required urgently in these circumstances in order to terminate the pregnancy and repair or remove the tube.

Bleeding after 28 weeks can be caused by the placenta

peeling away from the uterine wall before delivery. It will be accompanied by a continuous pain and shock, because the blood loss is internal too. This is an indication for ringing a hospital immediately because the baby is being deprived of oxygen, and the mother's life is also at risk. If abruptio placenta, as it is known, is diagnosed, the baby must be delivered immediately by caesarean section.

Another cause of bleeding in later pregnancy can be from placenta praevia, which is caused by the placenta developing in the lower part of the uterus so that it totally or partially blocks the cervix. Once the cervix starts to stretch in preparation for labour, the placenta can be torn from its site and painless, bright red bleeding takes place. Placenta praevia can be detected by ultrasound. If it is, a woman may be expected to spend the last months of pregnancy in hospital because the risk of a sudden, disastrous haemorrhage is high, and the baby has to be born by caesarean section. If the placenta only partially blocks the cervix, normal delivery is possible, although it must be in hospital. There is a homeopathic remedy for marginal placenta praevia — take Erigeron 3x three times a day until the problem has gone, perhaps three to four weeks.

Bleeding can also occur normally at the start of labour, quite heavily in some cases. If it is heavy enough to soak a pad, you should contact your midwife or hospital.

Homeopathic remedies

There are some very specific treatments for bleeding in pregnancy, depending on the cause and character of the bleeding. Everyone should take Arnica as soon as the bleeding starts.

Causes
- **From trauma** — Arnica and cinnamon; if there is a delay in getting the actual remedy you can make a tea from ground cinnamon as a temporary substitute.
- **From fright** — Aconite. If the fright has turned to shock, a state of near-paralysis or non-reaction, stupor or

even unconsciousness — Opium.
- **From anger or temper, even if it is not yours —** Chamomilla.
- **From exitement, agitation, manic states —** Cimicifuga.
- **From mental depression, shock, strain caused by sick-nursing** — Baptisia.
- **From debility** — Aletris Farinosa; Caulophyllum; China; Helonias; Secale.
- **If degeneration of the placenta is diagnosed —** Phosphorus.

Type of bleeding
Character of blood: dark, fluid — Secale
light, fluid — Millefolium
haemorrhage which will not stop — Thlapsi Bursa
intermittent, with spasmodic pains, wants fresh air — Pulsatilla
labour-like pains, no bleeding — Secale
pains from the back round the abdomen and down thighs, crampy, squeezing — Viburnum
partly clotted, with pains from small of back to pubis, worse from motion — Sabina
with pains from small of back to thighs, weak back, worse from motion — Kali Carbonicum
scanty, or long oozing, irregular pains with weakness and trembling — Caulophyllum

BREECH BABY

A baby is said to be in a breech position if it presents its bottom rather than its head — that is its bottom tries to be born first. The delivery of breech babies is becoming an

increasingly contentious issue. Formerly these children —
3 per cent of all babies at full-term — were delivered at
home by doctors or midwives experienced in breech
deliveries. Nowadays the skill is being lost so that in many
cases breech is an automatic indication for delivery by
caesarean section. The anxiety is that the baby's head
may be subject to sudden pressure after the rapid delivery
of the body, and that there is only a limited amount of
time in which to get the baby's head through the pelvis. If
you want to try having your breech baby vaginally, you
may have to search for a consultant or independent
midwife who is willing to help you. An upright, active birth
without an epidural is the best way to bring the baby
down.

Needless to say it is far more satisfactory to persuade
the baby to turn so that it is head-down well before birth
and there are a number of ways of attempting this. In fact
the baby only starts to become fixed at around 32 weeks
in a first pregnancy and at around 34 in subsequent ones,
so it is not worth worrying about its position before then,
unless you have had a breech baby before. You may
suspect your baby is breech if you can feel its hard round
head under your ribs, and you can get a sudden feeling of
urgency if the baby kicks you in the bladder. Once you are
certain that it is the wrong way up, start by giving gravity
a chance. The head is the heaviest part of the baby, and
inverting yourself, ideally head down in a pool swimming
for as long and as often as your can manage, should
provide a good opportunity for a shift of position. You can
practise a modified version of this exercise at home by
lying with your hips much higher than your head — either
on your back with a pile of cushions under your bottom
and the soles of your feet on the floor, or by kneeling on the
floor with your bottom in the air and your head resting on
your arms on the floor. Sleep with three or four pillows
under your bottom.

Try to relax completely and talk to the baby telling it
why you want it to move and visualising it head down. If
the baby's bottom has engaged you will need to make the

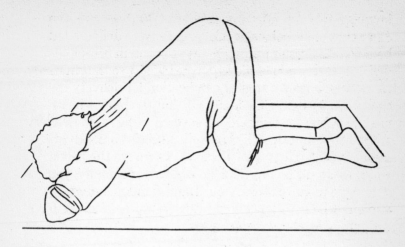

The knee-chest position

angle steeper. If the baby does turn late, you may feel it as a great, and possibly painful churning in your abdomen. Don't give up hope, babies have been known to turn at 40 weeks.

Homeopathic remedies
Try Pulsatilla 200 in two doses, two days apart in the 35th week. Pulsatilla is also good for altering a baby's position in labour. Alternatively consult a homeopath for an individual diagnosis and treatment.

Acupuncture
This has a good record of success in turning babies. The treatment should be started at 35 weeks and you can either visit a practitioner or try the technique — known as moxibustion — at home. It involves the burning of moxa or mugwort, a slow-burning herb, over the skin beside the nail of both little toes. If you can get moxa (available from the Acumedic Centre, see p. 177), make a small cone of it and light it with a joss stick so that it smoulders rather

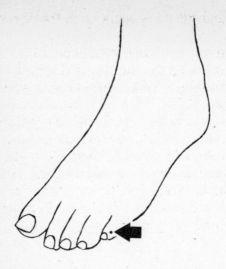

Acupressure point for turning malpositioned baby

than burns with a flame. If you cannot get moxa, you can hold a cigarette ¼ inch (5 mm) away from the skin. Allow it to warm, but not burn, your skin for 10 minutes on each little toe twice a day until the baby moves.

This treatment is useful for any malposition.

CONSTIPATION

This is a common complaint in pregnancy and occurs because the high levels of progesterone in the bloodstream act on the smooth muscles of the intestine to slow it down. You can improve the situation by altering your diet, taking more exercise and changing your posture while sitting. For the latter, try sitting on a tilted chair — the kind that keeps your back straight, so that your knees are lower than your hips.

Dietary changes include eating more fruit, vegetables, nuts and seeds, and dried fruit. Bran is not necessarily helpful as it can reduce iron absorption. It will also help to eat fibre-rich foods, such as lentils, oats and whole grains and to cut out refined carbohydrates. Red meat can cause constipation, and should be replaced in the diet with fish and poultry.

Dehydration can result in constipation; in this case it might be accompanied by a headache. This will be improved by drinking several pints of spring water or diluted fruit juice daily.

Some of the other causes of constipation include taking iron tablets, and drinking too much milk and tea. Try taking Floradix liquid instead of iron tablets (see p. 41–2), cutting down on dairy products and drinking herbal teas.

Chewing gum helps some sufferers. Others may find that psyllium seeds taken as 2 teaspoonful in water first thing in the morning improve matters.

Massage
Lying on your back, try stroking with the fingers of both hands down the midline of your stomach from your chest to your pubic bone, up either side to your armpits, over your breasts and down again. Repeat this 21 times.

Nutritional supplements
200 mg magnesium can help, especially if you have suffered from pre-menstrual syndrome. Also try taking 1–5 g vitamin C per day.

Homeopathic remedies
If your habits are sedentary, you have hard, dry stools and an inactive rectum so that even soft stools are passed with difficulty, take Alumina. If you feel as though the bowel movement is incomplete and it is worse away from home, try Lycopodium. For fruitless urging, obstinate constipation, you strain to pass a small amount and are irritable, take Nux Vomica. For obstinate constipation, no urging for days, prolonged straining, feeling of a ball in the rectum, the remedy is Sepia.

For constipation associated with piles which bleed and are painful, take Hydrastis.

If you are constipated and have a splitting headache, a dry mouth, feel thirsty and are irritable and want to keep still, take Bryonia.

Herbal remedy
Try drinking one cup of rhubarb root tea each night before going to bed. (See also Haemorrhoids, pp. 58–60.)

Acupuncture
Treatment provided by an acupuncturist can be very successful in dealing with the problem of constipation during pregnancy.

CRAMP

Sudden sharp pains in the feet or legs can be an indication of cramp, a condition which is common in pregnancy. There are quite a few remedies, some for immediate use, others long-term.

When cramp hits you, grab your toes and pull them towards your knees, or, get out of bed and stand at arm's length from the wall, with your palms flat against it. Keeping your feet flat on the floor, lean towards the wall and stay in this position until the cramp has gone. Alternatively you can pinch the area in between the root of your big toe and the one next to it, applying pressure firmly.

The other measures include getting up slowly in the morning, doing eye-rolling exercises first and being sure not to stretch out fully. You can try elevating the head of your bed or wearing an anklet of corks.

Nutritional supplements
Increase your calcium and magnesium intake by taking 6 Dolomite tablets per day. Also take a vitamin B-complex supplement daily. A teaspoonful of salt at tea-time can work wonders.

Aromatherapy
Hot foot baths with 10 drops of lavender oil can be very beneficial.

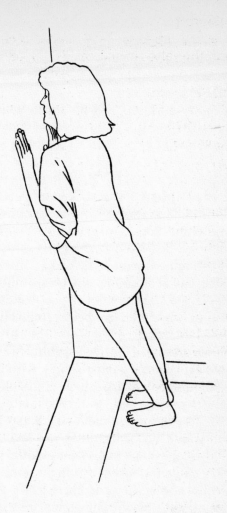

Muscle cramps in pregnancy

To relieve cramp in the feet or legs. Stand at arms length from the wall with your palms flat against it. Keeping your feet flat on the floor, lean towards the wall and stay in this position until the cramp is gone.

Herbal remedies
One or two glasses of cramp bark decoction daily may help.

Homeopathic remedies
Crush three pills of Mag Phos with a little warm water and sip as needed.

CYSTITIS

This unpleasant affliction can strike quite suddenly. It is caused by an inflammation of the bladder and results in a frequent and painful desire to urinate, even when the bladder is empty. Passing urine gives rise to a sensation of burning and stinging. It can be helped by drinking several pints of water, each containing one teaspoonful of sodium bicarbonate. If you start as soon as you feel the first twinge, a full-blown attack can be averted. The more you can drink the better.

Some people are particularly susceptible to cystitis and there is some evidence of a possible link with both thrush (see p. 78–80) and food allergies (see p. 154). If you suffer from cystitis frequently, you should see if either of these apply to you. For instance, a diet diary might show you a link between your attacks and what you eat.

You can also take steps to prevent an attack of cystitis by not getting chilled, wearing cotton underclothes and avoiding alcohol and sugary and spicy foods. Always urinate after making love. If home measures fail to clear up cystitis, it may be necessary to see your GP for some antibiotics, because of the risk of kidney infection. If you do need to take antibiotics, make sure that you take lactobacillus capsules at the same time, and/or eat plenty of live natural yoghurt.

Diet
A dietary regime which can help is as follows:

Day 1 Drink at least 4 pints (2.25 litres) of water with a teaspoonful of sodium bicarbonate per pint (600 ml) as above.

Make a soup with barley and vegetables and drink lots of the strained liquid.

Day 2 Include brown rice and vegetables and fish in the diet.

Day 3 Gradually return to a normal diet, avoiding meat until there have been no symptoms for 48 hours.

Homeopathy
Take Cantharis 6 three times a day for three days.

Aromatherapy
Try taking 2 drops of bergamot oil in a little alcohol.

Herbal remedies
You can take hot yarrow tea every two hours. This can also be combined with equal parts of bearberry and couchgrass to help ease the symptoms. Potter's Antitis tablets can also help some people, or try a teaspoonful of powdered marshmallow root in a cupful of boiling water. This forms a paste which can be sweetened with honey and taken three times a day before meals. This should help lessen the distressing burning sensation experienced when urinating.

FAINTING

This is common in early pregnancy, especially early in the morning or after a hot bath. It is due to progesterone acting on the smooth muscle and relaxing the muscles in the walls of your veins, with the result that blood pools in the legs and your brain becomes short of oxygen. The best remedy is to sit down with your head between your legs, and avoid rising suddenly if you are prone to faintness.

Dr Bach's Rescue Remedy — a few drops in water, or neat if you are outside — will help too.

Homeopathic remedies

For vertigo with falling to the left or backwards with a hot head, take Belladonna. With nausea, which is worse with travelling, outside or from emotions, take Cocculus. And for momentary loss of consciousness, which is worse outside or in the morning or after dinner, and better with resting, the remedy is Nux Vomica.

FEARFULNESS AND TENSION

Fear of labour is normal, especially if you have not been through it before. It may not bother you too much, you may just feel a lurch in the stomach when you realise that one way or another the baby has got to come out. You can use this anxiety positively, by making sure you feel comfortable about where you give birth, discussing it with your midwives, friends and at classes, making sure that you are fit for birth, eating well and by being well informed.

However anxiety can mount so that fears about the birth come to dominate your life, giving you sleepless nights and wretched days. This may be from fear of the unknown, or because you have some reason to think that there is something wrong with the baby, or because you have had problems with this pregnancy or in previous ones. This type of anxiety can be all-consuming and is not constructive. If it cannot be used to alter and improve matters, then determine either to forget it or to worry about it only between certain hours, say 9–10 am. Once you can do this, you may realise how even fretting for that length of time is fruitless.

Acupuncture can improve ante-natal depression. You might also be helped by hypnotherapy which would not only remove the anxiety, but could also teach you a technique for use as pain-relief in labour. Essential oils which can lift the spirits are jasmine, clary sage or ylang ylang. Put a few drops in your bath or float some in a saucer of warm water and inhale the aroma.

Fear and tension in labour can slow the labour down and may result in unnecessary intervention. It can help to be very open about the way you are feeling — a good midwife or partner will be able to encourage and reassure you. Tension builds up not only as a result of pain, but also because of the circumstances you may find yourself in, which is why it is important to have as much control of your situation as is possible. You will be taught conscious relaxation techniques at ante-natal classes and it is useful to use these to eliminate tension as far as possible.

Technique for relaxing

Find a comfortable position, in which you will be warm and free from distractions. Starting with your toes and working upwards, become aware of any tension in any part of your body and let it go. Focus on your feet, ankles, calves, thighs, pelvis, stomach, chest, shoulders, arms, hands, neck, face, jaw, mouth and scalp in turn. When you first practise this technique, you may find it easier to relax if you first tense each of the muscles for 10 seconds before letting go. Become aware of how those muscles feel when relaxed and take three slow breaths before you move on to the next group of muscles.

As you become more relaxed you will feel warmer, softer and heavier. If extraneous thoughts distract you, concentrate on pleasant images — imagine that you are lazing on a beach or in an idyllic garden or try to fill your whole mind with your favourite colour. As you become good at relaxing in this way, you can start to practise it in the sort of upright position which is best for labour.

Homeopathic remedies

For feelings of sudden fear, take Aconite. For a sensation of nervousness, take the tissue salt, Kali Phos. If you find yourself weeping frequently for no apparent reason, take Pulsatilla.

FORGETFULNESS

Pregnancy can have a temporary but devastating effect on your brain. Women speak of starting to talk and then forgetting completely what they were going to say, being unable to remember if they have started doing something, or not being able to recall the name of things. Although your faculties are not necessarily impaired, it does seem that the impact of pregnancy hormones can change your memory and personality so that you may react to things quite differently from the way you would if you were not pregnant.

The homeopathic remedy Nux Moschata may help, and you can try and be meticulous about making lists and keeping appointments, but the only real remedy is giving birth. It can still take a while after the baby is born before you really get your brain back.

HAEMORRHOIDS (PILES)

These are varicose veins around the anus and are caused by pressure on relaxed blood vessels. Piles usually start with irritation and itching inside the rectum and around the anal area. They become worse on straining and can eventually protrude. The condition can be very painful and there is no entirely satisfactory solution. Unfortunately, haemorrhoids do tend to get worse with subsequent pregnancies, but they do usually clear up after the birth. Occasionally however they are not present until after the birth when they appear suddenly and make the post-partum period very uncomfortable.

If you think that you are at risk from piles, do try to avoid becoming constipated (see p. 50) as the extra straining will exacerbate the problem. Use an ointment such as Nelson's Cream for Haemorrhoids available from health shops, or Anusol from a chemists to relieve the discomfort. Apply the cream after every bowel movement and at night. It comes with a special applicator so that you can insert the ointment into the rectum. Minimise straining by using a squatting position on the toilet. This can be done by stacking magazines either side of the loo. Pelvic floor exercises, concentrating on tightening the muscles around the anus, may help.

Put your feet up as much as you can, and try to rest with your bottom higher than your head. Piles which protrude can be pushed back very gently with a finger. It may help to soften them first by sitting in a bath.

If you have a tendency to piles, do not practise squatting, except in the position where you are lying on your back with your legs up against the wall.

If haemorrhoids remain prolapsed or if one becomes thrombosed, you will need to seek medical help.

Homeopathic remedies

For piles with a sore, raw feeling, take Hamamamelis. For blind (internal) piles with back pain and constipation, take Calc Fluor. If they come on suddenly and are acute, inflamed and make you feel restless and are worse with warmth, take Aconite. If they give rise to a stinging pain, are worse with backache and lying down, take Belladonna. If they are itching, burning and oozing perhaps with obstinate constipation or painless diarrhoea, the remedy is Sulphur. For very sore, protruding, bleeding, hot piles that are better with cold water, and cause a bearing down feeling in the rectum, take Aloe. Ainsworth, the homeopathic pharmacy, will make up suppositories to treat piles if you contact them by phone and describe the problem (address p. 181).

Herbal remedies

Take garlic perles, 1–6 per day (the one-a-day strength). Insert a peeled clove of garlic into the rectum at night. An infusion of pilewort three times a day or Potter's Pileabs may also help relieve the symptoms. Another possibility is to apply live yoghurt to the piles.

Aromatherapy

Cypress oil can shrink piles. Put a few drops in a

washing-up bowl full of warm water and sit in it for as long as you are comfortable.

HEADACHES

Unfortunately headaches are not uncommon in pregnancy, especially in the first few weeks. If you cannot avoid using pain killers, paracetamol is preferable to aspirin. There are, however, other very effective ways of easing a headache which do not involve taking drugs.

Aromatherapy
Rub a few drops of lavender oil on to your temples. For a sick headache, a drop of peppermint oil can be taken on a lump of sugar.

A compress can be made by soaking a cloth in half a pint (300 ml) of water to which six drops each of lavender and peppermint oil have been added. Lie down and put the cloth over your forehead. Rest is the best cure whenever possible.

Herbal remedies
Try poppyhead tea or an infusion of equal parts of balm, lavender and meadowsweet. Another remedy is to drop two cloves into a cup of tea, and allow them to infuse before drinking.

Biochemic tissue salts
Combination F is for migraine and nervous headaches.

Acupuncture
Headache in pregnancy is seen as being caused by a deficiency in the body, and the site of the headache indicates the type of deficiency, eg a headache on the top of the head means a problem in the liver. All types of pregnancy headache are treatable by acupuncture. You may be able to treat yourself with acupressure — see Julian Kenyon's book *Acupressure Techniques*.

Nutritional Supplements

Zinc — 25 mg per day — can have a wonderful effect on the type of headache you have when you start the day feeling as if you have a hangover.

IMPORTANT — headache, together with disturbance of vision, such as seeing flashing lights, raised blood pressure and severe fluid retention, can be a symptom of pre-eclampsia, a disease of the second half of pregnancy which if left can develop into toxaemia which is life-threatening (see under Hypertension). Contact medical help if you get a severe headache which cannot be relieved with painkillers.

HEARTBURN

Heartburn is caused by the action of progesterone relaxing the valve at the upper end of the stomach so that the acid contents of the stomach can pass back into the oesphagus. The condition is made worse by the growing baby pushing your stomach upwards. The problem is relieved by delivery, but if you suffer from the unpleasant burning sensation in the chest that is heartburn, you will want a remedy well before then. Some general remedies include avoiding fatty, spicy and acid foods, and alcohol and coffee. The best advice is to eat very small meals often, being sure to chew well and slowly. Also avoid bending or lying flat — it may help to sleep propped up, and perhaps put a brick under the head end of the bed. It is best to avoid antacids which are available on prescription or over the counter, because although they work initially, the stomach tends to increase its acid output to try and counter-act the alkalinity. They also contain a lot of aluminium hydroxide which can interfere with the absorption of certain nutrients and harm the fetus. Milk, too, works well but can have a rebound effect and increase the acid reflux.

Herbal remedies

1 teaspoon of slippery elm bark powder mixed with honey or hot water neutralises the acid and soothes the stomach.

Or drink aniseed or fennel tea as your daily beverage and try infusions of peppermint, meadowsweet or chamomile to remedy heartburn. Try chewing blanched almonds, dried papaya, or even washed orange peel as these could help too.

Homeopathic remedies
For heartburn and indigestion linked with thrush, take Nat Phos 6x tissue salt. With more definite flatulence and distension which is worse after eating, take Carbo Veg. If you have indigestion which feels like a stone in your stomach and have bitter eructations, take Nux Vomica. If you have heartburn and dyspepsia after meals and are not thirsty, and it is made much worse by eating fatty things, take Pulsatilla.

Aromatherapy
Maggie Tisserand in her book *Aromatherapy for Women* recommends one drop of sandalwood oil on the tongue. She says that peppermint or rose may help too.

HEAVY SWELLING (OEDEMA)

Some swelling of legs, hands and feet is common during pregnancy. Excessive swelling, which is very uncomfortable, may be reduced by stimulation of the lymphatic drainage system. Try applying constant pressure to a point in the muscle above each breast on the side nearest your armpit. If you feel around you should find a spot which is particularly tender. Simultaneously pressing and rubbing it will probably feel sore, but if done properly daily can reduce fluid retention.

Carpal Tunnel Syndrome
Oedema sometimes leads to compression of a large nerve at the wrist. This results in pain and numbness in the fingers, and can lead to you dropping things. Vitamin B6 up to 200 mg peal daily in a B complex sometimes helps.

HERPES

If you suffer from herpes include vitamin B12 (as a complex) with brewer's yeast in your diet. Use acidophulus capsules as pessaries and take them orally. Apply goldenseal (hydrastis) tincture locally and use an ice cube locally at the first sign of an outbreak. It is best to consult a homeopath for constitutional treatment, but Hepar Sulph 30 and Variolinum 30 once daily until there is an improvement should help. Ring Ainsworths for a remedy called Herpes pro genitalis.

HYPERTENSION (HIGH BLOOD PRESSURE)

Technically hypertension exists when your blood pressure has risen so that the diastolic pressure has risen 20 or more points above your normal pregnancy blood pressure, ie if your blood pressure in early pregnancy was 120/70 then it is unsatisfactorily high if it reaches 140/90. The normal range in pregnancy is from 90/50 to 130/80. The upper figure — the systolic — denotes the pressure generated by your heart as it pumps blood round your body. The lower pressure — known as the diastolic — indicates the pressure in your arteries when the heart is at rest and this is the figure which is of most significance because a large increase in diastolic pressure means a reduction in the supply of blood and oxygen to the baby, and that you are at risk of developing pre-eclampsia.

Pre-eclampsia, which can become toxaemia of pregnancy, is a disease exclusive to the second half of pregnancy. Its cause is not fully known, although it is thought to be immunological. It is experienced by 12 per cent of first-time mothers and only 4 per cent of those having subsequent babies. If untreated it can lead to severe convulsions in the mother and the death of the baby. A rise in blood pressure together with protein in the urine and fluid retention leading to a large weight gain constitute pre-eclampsia. It is a condition which can start quite suddenly, so the warning signs must be taken very seriously. These include:

- severe headaches which cannot be relieved by painkillers
- visual disturbances, like seeing flashing lights
- abdominal pain
- considerable swelling

If, however, your blood pressure is raised and you have no other signs of pre-eclampsia, you will probably be keen to find ways of getting it down, because otherwise you will be expected to rest while feeling perfectly fit. Moreover high blood pressure is one of the indications for induction of labour.

Eating well is of course important, although there are opposing theories about this. One, promoted by the American Dr Tom Brewer, states that pre-eclampsia is a disease of malnutrition and that it can be prevented by eating a high-protein diet with salt to taste. Another, maintains that blood pressure can be reduced by fasting on a diet of water melon and brown rice and then once it is back to normal avoiding red meat, spicy foods and alcohol and eating plenty of raw fruit and vegetables. Cut down on salt and drink six to eight glasses of pure spring water daily.

Nutritional supplements

Take a B-complex supplement that includes 50 mg of Vitamin B6 daily.

Also take 6 Dolomite tablets daily to increase calcium and magnesium intake.

Herbal remedies

Take garlic perles, between 2–10 daily, or eat several cloves of raw garlic. Try dandelion infusion at least twice daily. You can also eat raw or cooked dandelion leaves as well. Take celery in any form, as stalks, juice or as seeds in celery salt or try celeriac. Over-ripe cucumber is said to be useful too.

Alternatively, try ¼–1 teaspoonful cayenne three times a day taken in orange juice or yoghurt as a normaliser for blood pressure. Self-Heal Herbs sell a Circulation Formula which is designed to restore normal circulation (see p. 180 for the address).

Acupuncture

Acupuncture can effectively reduce essential hypertension, that is chronically raised pressure that gives a high reading in early pregnancy.

Homeopathic remedies

Kali Chlor is the remedy for hypertension although it is probably best to consult a homeopath.

One last theory that appears to work well is that ¼ of a tablet of aspirin taken daily can prevent pre-eclampsia in susceptible women. If you are at risk, it would be worth discussing this with your midwife or obstetrician.

INSOMNIA

This is very common in later pregnancy for a number of reasons: it may be hard to get comfortable in bed, you may have to get up to go to the loo several times a night, or be disturbed by the baby kicking and your bed may suddenly seem too hard. If you usually sleep on your stomach, trying to get to sleep can be miserable.

The practical steps that you can take are: use extra pillows under the bulge or to prop you up, have a bucket at the bedside, and perhaps sleep in another bed. Many couples find that neither get much rest in a double bed at this stage. It can help to get up and go into another room, or make a drink of honey and lemon.

Sometimes anxiety can prevent you sleeping, either by stopping you getting to sleep or by causing you to wake in the night, perhaps after dreadfully vivid nightmares about the baby or labour. You may find discussing your anxieties with friends, midwife or NCT teacher helps. Other worries can be tackled by taking an objective view of your problems and seeing how you would advise a friend in the same situation.

Practising relaxation techniques, cutting out any daytime sleep that you may be getting and taking regular daily exercise can give you a better night.

Acupuncture

Acupuncture can have a very beneficial effect on sleeplessness at any time.

Homeopathic remedies

Nelson's Noctura tablets which are a combination remedy can be very effective. Or try Cocculus when you have difficulty in getting back to sleep again or Coffea Crud. when sleepless from excitement or too much coffee, when pain is unsupportable and too many thoughts are filling your mind.

Herbal remedies

You can try infusions made from any of the following herbs: hops, passion flower, elderflower, Californian poppy, or valerian. You could also try using them in baths. To do this you pour 2 pints (1.2 litres) of boiling water on to one or two handfuls of the herb. Allow it to stand for half an hour, strain, then pour into a hot bath. Avena Sativa compound from Weleda works well. Take 10–20 drops in water half an hour before bed.

Aromatherapy

Massage at bedtime is soothing and relaxing and can help you sleep. Try putting a drop of neroli oil or clary sage on the edge of your pillow, or using them in a massage oil.

METALLIC TASTE IN THE MOUTH

You may find that you are plagued by an ever-present unusual taste of metal in your mouth. It tends to be a symptom of early pregnancy.

If it is a strong, slimy taste with a lot of saliva, try the homeopathic remedy Cuprum Met 6. If it is sweetish with coppery saliva try Merc Sol 6.

Herbal remedies include mouth washes with fennel, rosemary and rhyme. Weleda make one that contains extract of myrrh and krameria — the Peruvian toothbrush plant. A nutritional supplement of zinc, 25 mg per day, if you are not already taking it, should help.

MISCARRIAGE

As many as one in two pregnancies fail to go to full-term. The majority of those lost are in the very earliest stages of pregnancy, perhaps even before the first period is missed or in the days afterwards. Women often suspect this when they experience symptoms of pregnancy and then have a late period, one which might be particularly heavy or painful.

Later on, miscarriage may be signalled by bleeding from the vagina together with contractions of the uterus. Even bleeding alone can be very frightening and upsetting. Not much can be done conventionally to help, but you will be advised to go to bed and rest. This may help and at least you will feel that you are doing everything you can to save the baby, although there is no evidence to show that this alters the miscarriage rate, and healthy babies are born to mothers who have not been able to rest while bleeding. Miscarriage is more likely when there is bright red bleeding, there are contractions and the neck of the cervix is open.

At least 50 per cent of miscarriages are due to nature discarding a fetus with abnormalities. The process of fertilisation and subsequent pregnancy is enormously complex and inevitably does not always take place perfectly. However you are more likely to be unhappy that your baby has not survived than to be consoled by the thought that it might have had an abnormality.

If you know that you are pregnant and the bleeding and contractions continue until spontaneous abortion (as miscarriage is technically known) takes place, you may find that you know when the fetus has been passed. However, it is not always evident even when a miscarriage is complete, because sometimes the fetus is re-absorbed. If the miscarriage occurs early in the pregnancy the fetus can look like a lump of hard, whitish tissue. A later miscarriage produces a fetus which is recognisably human. Ultrasound has a place here, as it can be used to tell whether or not the fetus is still alive despite the bleeding. If you do miscarry, it can be helpful to keep everything that comes away (known as the products of conception), so that a doctor can see if any tissue has been retained. If it has, you might need a D and C (dilatation and curettage) to completely clear the uterus. You will generally be admitted to hospital when you miscarry, although women who have miscarried before sometimes find they are happier if they stay at home and manage everything themselves.

If you are rhesus negative and your partner is not, it is important to have an anti-D injection following a birth, a miscarriage or even a threatened miscarriage, in order that you do not risk developing anti bodies to rhesus positive blood which might harm subsequent children.

There are some good alternative treatments for a threatened miscarriage, although it is important to note that such treatments will not work to retain a damaged fetus.

Acupuncture
With bleeding in early pregnancy an acupuncturist will treat you twice within a 24–36 hour period, which should stop the bleeding. He will then correct the deficiency and see you weekly for about a month. You may be given Moxa (a slow burning herb used to apply heat to acupuncture points) to use at home, and you may also be advised about diet and rest.

Herbal remedies
Any of the following herbal remedies might help.

- False unicorn root (helonias), ½ oz (15 g) to a pint (600 ml) of water, boiled and simmered gently for 15

minutes. Drink copiously. Alternatively try 2–3 drops of the tincture, three times a day.
- Wild yam root, take 2–4 fl oz (50–120 ml) of infusion every half an hour. The tincture is said to be less successful and may cause vomiting. Take 10 drops every half an hour.
- Lobelia tincture, no more than 15 drops in a small glass of water every 15 minutes as needed.

Nutritional supplements
- Vitamin E, up to 2,000 IUs per day
- Zinc, 25 mg
- Manganese chloride or amino-chelate, 10–20 mg
- Essential fatty acids, 1–4 g Efamol per day.

Osteopathy
A cranial osteopath can help prevent a miscarriage by working viscerally, through the abdominal wall, to calm down the contractions of the uterus.

Massage
A gentle massage can help to bring down the heart rate and open veins and arteries so they can work to capacity. Make a massage oil from 15 drops of clary sage in 2 oz (50 ml) of olive oil to help relieve the pain and anxiety, and use it with some of the massage techniques on pp. 96–7.

Homeopathy
See pp. 45–7. Treatment for an incomplete miscarriage is Secale Pyrogen. For Septicaemia with feverishness and evil-smelling discharge Pyrogen. There are several remedies for those who do not recover completely afterwards; consult a homeopath.

Alcohol
As a short-term measure, alcohol will inhibit or slow down contractions.

Bach flower remedy

Take a few drops of Rescue Remedy (see p. 8) in a glass of water. This is particularly good for dealing with shock at the first sight of bleeding.

If you have experienced bleeding in pregnancy it is best to avoid intercourse for at least two weeks after the bleeding has stopped. If you miscarry more than once it may be best to avoid sex until 16 weeks of pregnancy.

MISCARRIAGE, RECURRENT

Miscarrying repeatedly is very distressing indeed. Even one miscarriage causes you to doubt your body and feel anxiety about subsequent pregnancies, but when it keeps on happening your feelings of hopelessness and despair can be quite overwhelming. There are orthodox treatments, such as hormone injections, running a stitch round the cervix if weakness is causing it to open prematurely, and other newer and successful techniques. The Miscarriage Association (see p. 183) is able to provide details, and also self-help and support when needed.

Alternatives are well worth considering for this problem. Conventionally you are only deemed to have a problem after a third or subsequent miscarriage, but you may well want to try to find a solution before you reach this point.

Acupuncture

Nearly all the conditions for recurrent miscarriage are treatable by acupuncture.

Liz was in her late thirties and had had two miscarriages at 10 and 12 weeks. She visited an acupuncturist who diagnosed too little blood and a tendency to flush everything out. She was treated and given advice about her diet. Her recurrent headaches ceased and she had no more attacks of herpes. Within two months she was pregnant and with further treatment carried the baby to term. When the baby was overdue, her labour was started by acupuncture. She felt in the peak of health throughout pregnancy and gave birth to a healthy boy.

Nutritional supplements
Take the supplements recommended for a first miscarriage for at least a month prior to conception, and follow the pre-conception advice in chapter 3.

Herbal remedies
Take one or two cups of black haw root tea daily from the start of the pregnancy. Another recommendation is to take three drops of the tincture of false unicorn root four or five times a day from a month before conception until 14 weeks of the pregnancy.

Homeopathy
If there is a tendency to abort at the second or third month, it would be well worth consulting a homeopath.

MORNING SICKNESS

Morning sickness — which can, in fact, occur at any time of the day and sometimes night — is absolutely miserable. It can vary from intermittent mild nausea to permanent nausea and constant vomiting. It may even consist of sudden vomiting without nausea. In general it is limited to a period starting any time from days or weeks after conception until 12–14 weeks, although some unfortunate women have it throughout pregnancy. Even knowing that it is likely to end is not much help if you feel as if you are dying and you have only just got a positive pregnancy test. It is more common in those expecting their first child, a girl or more than one baby. Although it makes you feel appalling, be assured that the retching will not damage the baby, nor does it seem to be deprived by your only managing to keep down a little food.

There are a lot of suggestions about what might help this unpleasant condition. If one remedy does not work, try another. Start by looking at ways in which changing your routine might improve the problem.

- Have a glass of apple juice beside your bed, so that you can sip some in the night and have a drink first thing in the morning.
- If possible have tea and dry biscuits brought to you in bed, and get up gradually.
- Eat small, bland, easily prepared meals frequently.
- Rest as much as possible, in bed whenever there is the chance.
- Take regular exercise — a brisk walk can help alleviate feelings of nausea.

The supplements which may help, if you are not already taking them, are:

Vitamin B6, 10–100 mg per day
Magnesium, 200–400 mg per day
Zinc sulphate, 25 mg per day
Brewer's yeast, 2 heaped teaspoonfuls mixed with milk and mashed banana
Vitamin K injections are said to help

Herbal remedies

Ginger has a good reputation as a remedy for sickness of any kind. It can be taken in any form, as tablets, a few drops of essence or tincture, crystallised, ginger beer or as an infusion made with fresh shredded root or ordinary powdered ginger.

Other herbs which may help if taken as infusions are: chamomile, peppermint, hops, lemon balm, meadowsweet, black horehound, gentian, raspberry leaf. Peppermint can also be taken as one drop of essential oil on a sugar lump. Biostrath Elixir will restore your appetite and replace missing nutrients.

Homeopathic therapies

Think about your symptoms and how you are feeling generally, then see how they equate with those given below. The remedy that describes your symptoms most accurately is the one to try.

Ipecac — constant nausea and/or vomiting which is not relieved by vomiting; clean tongue; may be irritable and probably suffer from loss of appetite; feel worse lying down.

Sepia — feelings of nausea are worse in the mornings; can't bear the smell or sight of food or cooking; there is no loss of appetite, and indeed symptoms may be relieved by food; may experience an empty feeling in stomach and possibly feel depressed or indifferent.

Ant. Tart. — spasmodic vomiting of undigested food and mucus immediately after eating; exhaustion or collapse. May be worse in the evening and better from sitting upright.

Nux Vomica — spasmodic vomiting after breakfast; bitter taste in the stomach; stomach feels as though it contains a heavy weight; may be constipated and be irritable.

Arg. Nit. — nausea and vomiting with flatulence; experience a craving for sweet things; want fresh air; worse from heat and may be anxious or panicky.

Aromatherapy
The essential oils which may make you feel better are: lavender, chamomile, rose.

Acupuncture
Acupuncture works well on the special points for stopping sickness, or you could buy a Sea Band marketed for sea-sickness which applies pressure to one of the points (available from Novafon Ltd, see p. 184 for the address). Alternatively, you can make your own by strapping a pebble tightly on to the inside of your wrist, three fingers down from your first wrist crease and in between your two tendons.

Osteopathy
Consider this if bending over a sink or the loo damages your spine. Problems in the dorsal spine can affect the

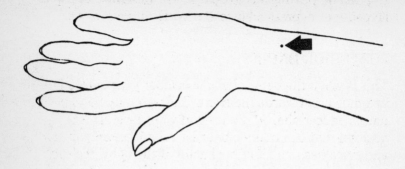

Acupunture point to stop morning sickness

Apply pressure to a point on your wrist, three fingers down from the wrist crease, in between the two tendons.

vagus nerve leading to the stomach which when irritated can cause vomiting.

NASAL CONGESTION

Some women seem to have a blocked nose throughout pregnancy, due to relaxed blood vessels in the nose caused by the increase in progesterone. Unfortunately there is not much that can be done about this because it is part of the general facial swelling, although putting a few drops of eucalyptus or peppermint oil onto a handkerchief may help. Rosemary oil in an essential oil burner can clear the air and make breathing easier.

Women are often concerned that a cold will prevent them using breathing techniques in labour. Quite often the nose clears during labour, though the cold returns after the birth.

NOSE BLEEDS

These are also common in pregnancy because of the increased amount of blood in your system. They can be stopped by putting a cold compress containing a drop of lavender or cypress oil over the bridge of your nose.

POSTERIOR BABIES

This is when the baby's back is against your back so that its limbs are towards the front. One sign may be that you have a saucer-shaped dip around your navel. It is a position that can make labour longer and more painful and gives rise to a lot of backache. If the baby does not turn during the course of labour — most do — it can mean that forceps are needed.

To try and shift the baby, spend a lot of time on all fours; the weight of the baby's head should swing the rest of it round. Use this position in labour too. Crawling may help.

PREMATURE LABOUR

Going into labour at any time before about 37 weeks can be very frightening. You may realise that labour is starting if you are getting regular contractions which may feel like tightenings of your abdomen, aches in your back or at the front, or stronger versions of the Braxton Hicks contractions that you may already be used to. Premature labour can also start with bleeding or rupture of the membranes. If you are not due for a long time yet, it might not occur to you that this could be labour and you might think that you have got a stomach upset or be suffering from indigestion.

However if you think you might be in labour, call your midwife or doctor or hospital and have a stiff drink — alcohol can inhibit contractions. If you are certain that you are in labour, call an ambulance because premature labour can be quite rapid and premature babies do need hospital facilities. If the baby is going to be very premature, ie less than 30 weeks, it would be as well if possible to get to a hospital with specialist intensive care facilities even if you are not booked there. It can be easier to move a very early baby before it is born, rather than afterwards. If you are travelling to hospital trying to prevent an imminent birth, try to adopt the knee-chest position where you are on your knees with your bottom high in the air and your head is on your crossed arms. If it is available you could try taking motherwort tincture — as much as is needed to stop contractions.

In some women painful, regular contractions occur for varying lengths of time throughout pregnancy. If this happens to you, check that your cervix is not dilating, then rest with a hot water bottle to ease the pain. You can also try small amounts of a decoction of false unicorn root — ½ oz (15 g) to a pint (600 ml) of water, simmered for 15 minutes. Other remedies include taking a decoction of cramp bark or an infusion of black horehound and ladies' slipper. Wild Mexican yam is useful for pains in pregnancy.

Homeopathic remedies
Treat the cause, see the remedies for miscarriage, on p. 46. If the membranes have ruptured, take Arnica. When the pains begin, take Sabina.

It is encouraging to know that membranes which rupture prematurely, often at the time of a growth spurt at 32 weeks, can heal over if you rest.

If travelling long distances by car remember to stop and walk around every couple of hours or so. One Devon obstetrician reports unusually high numbers of premature births in women who have driven to Devon from the North of England without a break.

PRESSURE OF THE BABY'S HEAD ON YOUR PELVIS

The baby's head can press on nerves in your pelvis, causing discomfort. This usually passes as the baby shifts position, but occasionally they get stuck in an awkward position and it becomes a real problem. The homeopathic remedy for this is Bellis Perennis 6. Acupuncture and osteopathy could also help or you could try a pelvic rock. This is done by sitting back on your heels and tipping your pelvis back and forth. This may move the baby and it can also be useful to give a bit of extra bladder room if you are going out.

SACRO-ILIAC JOINT PAIN

This can be an agonising pain caused by the loosening of the ligaments allowing the two sides of the sacro-iliac joint to move and grate together. It is felt low down on the back just under the dimples above the buttocks. It causes pain on turning over in bed, climbing stairs and can be quite crippling. Osteopathy is the best treatment.

SCIATIC NERVE PAIN

This is a pain which radiates down your thigh and can cause great discomfort. It can be improved by an osteopath or chiropractor or by massage with Nelson's Rhus Tox cream.

Aromatherapy
Treat as an inflammatory condition and rub in oil of lavender and/or wintergreen. You could also apply a poultice.

SKIN DISCOLOURATION

Women sometimes develop a discolouration of the skin on the face in pregnancy, traditionally known as a butterfly mask. It can appear as a brownish stain covering the nose and parts of the cheeks. Generally the discolouration fades slowly after the birth. There does not seem to be much that can be done about it, although it has been suggested that PABA, para-aminobenzoic acid, may help. This can be taken as a supplement of up to 500 mg per day. It is also found naturally in wheatgerm, whole grains, liver, mushrooms, fresh fruit and vegetables.

It is usual for a brown line to appear on the abdomen from the top of the pubic hair line to the navel.

THRUSH OR CANDIDA ALBICANS

Thrush is generally understood to mean a vaginal infection which results in a white curdy discharge and intense itching which can make your skin very sore. It is caused by a yeast which is present in everyone, but which, on occasion, becomes out of control.

It is more common in pregnancy because the fungus thrives on the sweeter, moister condition of the vagina in pregnancy. It is generally treated with anti-fungal pessaries which treat the symptoms, but may not prevent a recurrence. If you get thrush frequently, you should consider whether you might be one of the many people that suffer from systemic candida. This is a condition where the immune system has become weakened so that candida is able to gain control of the body. This can occur following the use of antibiotics, the pill or steroids. Even eating meat that has been treated by antibiotics can trigger the condition. Symptoms can include: recurrent thrush or cystitis, endometriosis, athlete's foot, allergies, abdominal bloating, diarrhoea or constipation, pre-menstrual syndrome, depression, lethargy, poor memory, muscle aches, tingling, numbness or burning, aches and swellings in the joints, menstrual cramps, spots before the eyes and loss of libido. You may be a sufferer if you are badly affected by the smell of perfumes, tobacco smoke or chemicals, or if you crave sweet foods, bread or alcohol.

Candida is treatable, but it may require several months on a diet which avoids the yeasty and sugary foods that candida lives off. Ideally this should be before you become pregnant, but it can be done while you are pregnant provided you are very careful to balance your diet. The process can be speeded up by taking supplements which encourage the growth of healthy intestinal flora and create an environment that is hostile to candida. Oral Nystatin can be prescribed by your doctor which will speed the process, but this is best taken before you become pregnant.

The foods that should be avoided are: bread, cakes, biscuits, anything in breadcrumbs, mushrooms, soya sauce, sour cream, black tea, all cheeses, citric acid, dried fruit, alcohol, malted products, vinegars, anything with sugar in, smoked or preserved meats or fish, nuts that have not been freshly cracked. Fresh fruit should be avoided for the first three weeks. Do not take any nutritional supplements that are not stated to be yeast-free.

It is quite probable that you may feel worse as the candida starts to die off, but this feeling will pass after several days.

You can help yourself still further by eating live, natural yoghurt, taking capsules of lactobacillus daily (available in a non-dairy form for those allergic to milk) and perhaps taking some acidophilus or Probion. Take two or more garlic perles daily as well as a zinc supplement (25 mg daily)

Remedies for a current attack of thrush
First insert two Probion tablets into the vagina. Try also to eat live natural yoghurt. You can dab yoghurt directly to the afflicted parts too. Take at least three garlic perles twice a day and eat raw garlic if you can manage it. Also insert a clove of peeled garlic into your vagina. Drink raspberry leaf tea instead of tea and completely cut out any form of sugar in your diet, including alcohol. A poultice made from slippery elm bark powder and water, backed with muslin and applied to the affected part can be soothing.

Babies can be born with candida (see p. 175) and thus may inherit a weakened immune system.

Homeopathic remedies
Nat Phos 6x tissue salt may help or try Candida 30. Also try eating sprouted wheat fresh or as tablets daily.

Aromatherapy

This is Maggie Tisserand's receipt for a vaginal douche for thrush from her book *Aromatherapy for Women*. A douche is absolutely CONTRA-INDICATED in pregnancy, but it can help to sit in a washing-up bowl of the liquid: place 2 drops rose, 4 drops lavender, and 2 drops bergamot in 2 pints (1.2 litres) of warm water and stir well.

Another remedy is to try sitting in bowls of hot and cold water alternately, adding a teaspoonful of the anti-fungal thyme and tea tree oils to each.

TIREDNESS

Tiredness is closely allied with motherhood. It is an extremely common side effect of early pregnancy and many women spend the first three months desperate for extra sleep. Towards the end of pregnancy, it is usual to sleep badly because of the difficulty in getting comfortable and because you may need to get up several times a night to go to the loo. This can seem like an unwelcome training programme for the nights following the birth, when frequent night feeds will cause you to be more tired than you ever thought possible.

Unfortunately, the best remedy — more sleep — is often the one that is least available. At any stage it is a good idea to cut down on your activities whenever possible, so that you can sleep or rest more. This may mean you need to make some radical changes in your lifestyle and perhaps accept that becoming a parent does make a difference to the way you live. In the early stages of pregnancy you might have to go out less or reduce your working hours; later on you may also need to have a rest during the day. If you are completely exhausted as a new mother, you should abandon everything that is not essential to survival. This can be particularly difficult because of the pressures upon you to cope and also because you will feel that your individuality is being lost if all you can do is cater for the baby and yourself. Anaemia can also cause tiredness (see pp. 41–2).

Taking oil of evening primrose can help to counter the effects of fatigue. Try taking up to six 500 mg capsules a day.

Coffee, tea, chocolate and colas and sweet foods can make tiredness worse by providing an instant energy boost which is followed by an energy low. Consequently, it is best to avoid such foods and drinks if you are feeling very tired.

VARICOSE VEINS

Varicose veins can appear for the first time in pregnancy, and often get worse in subsequent pregnancies. They may appear in your legs or vulva and cause considerable discomfort by aching and itching. They can be apparent as bulging, bluish veins under the skin or may ache without being especially visible. The right leg is often the worst affected.

You can help yourself by putting on support tights *before* you get out of bed in the morning — this gives the veins support before gravity increases the pressure of blood within them. Walking is helpful, too, because it aids the return of blood to your heart. Squatting is not recommended. Instead lie on your back with your legs up the wall. In fact try to lie with your legs higher than your head whenever possible.

Vulval varicose veins may be more comfortable if you wear a sanitary pad in well-fitting pants. Try soaking it in cypress oil and water first. If there is no improvement the veins may need to be cauterised.

Aromatherapy
Massaging the veins gently with diluted cypress oil will help to shrink them. Also try adding a few drops of lemon and cypress oils to your bath.

Nutritional supplements
Take extra vitamin E 300–600 IUs per day, together with 1–6 garlic perles.

Homeopathic remedies

For aching legs that feel bruised and strained, take
Arnica. If your legs are weary and feel as if you can't walk,
take Bellis Perennis. If you have varicose veins as well
and your legs feel bruised and sore and congested, take
Hamamelis.

8.
THE BIRTH

The questions that you will want answered in late
pregnancy are — how and when will labour start, what
will it be like, will I be able to cope, will I let myself down?
It is impossible to make accurate predictions about
anything to do with childbirth. You should remember this
when someone tells you that you will have had the baby by
next week or lunchtime, or that it will be a difficult or easy
birth, or that the baby will be huge or tiny. You can only go
by the way that you feel. It is better to avoid asking for
estimates about any of these things, because people are
notoriously wrong, and you may be basing your course of
action on a guess.

However, here are some guidelines that may enable you
to find the answers to your questions about your own
labour.

THE INDICATIONS THAT LABOUR IS STARTING

Labour starts when the level of progesterone in the body
falls and the level of oestrogen rises. This can result in any
of the following symptoms, but it is important to
remember that you can often seem to be starting only for
all the signs to die away for another few days or even
weeks. You will feel less frustrated if you play down early
symptoms so that there is the minimum of fuss when it
turns out not to be labour at all.

Weight loss
A decrease in the amount of amniotic fluid can mean that
you lose about 2–3 lbs (1–1.5 kg) in the last few days
before labour. You may find that you can feel your baby
more distinctly through your abdominal wall.

The baby moves less

Towards the end of the pregnancy the baby has much less room to move and you will feel fewer kicks than you did, say at 32 weeks. In the last few days the baby may slow down still more. If it kicks less than ten times in twelve hours, speak to your midwife, doctor or hospital. They will want to monitor the baby, probably on a cardiotocograph or belt monitor.

Nesting instinct

This is the famous urge to rush round preparing your nest for the imminent arrival of the baby — for some reason it often seems to manifest itself in a desire to clean the oven! If you are affected by this instinct, make sure that you conserve your energy so that you are not completely exhausted by the time contractions start.

Diarrhoea or stomach upset

Many women report having to make numerous trips to the loo at the start of their labours. It seems to be nature's way of clearing the bowel so that a full rectum does not impede the baby's passage down the birth canal.

Feeling different

Sometimes women wake feeling different, it may be better or worse than usual. It has been described as feeling 'fluey', 'irritable', 'extra uncomfortable' or even 'really brilliantly well'.

Show

This is the mucus plug which fills the cervix during pregnancy and acts as a barrier between the vagina and the baby and the bag of membranes. As your cervix changes shape at the very start of labour, the plug is loosened and comes away so that you may find it in your pants or on the loo paper. It can appear like a lump of sticky, clear jelly which may be streaked with blood making it appear pink, although some women find that theirs is quite loose and runny. Occasionally there is blood with it caused by the membranes becoming detached from the wall of the uterus. If it is bright red and enough to soak a pad, call your midwife or hospital.

Rupture of the membranes

This is one of the things which can cause anxiety. The majority of membranes (the tough bag which contains the baby and the amniotic fluid which surrounds it) rupture at home, but women do worry that it will happen when they are out. This isn't as embarrassing as it might seem and no-one will think that you have wet yourself. In fact most people will be unlikely to notice.

When the waters go, it may be with an audible pop or ping and a feeling that something has 'gone'. It will be followed by a gush or a trickle depending on the size of the rupture and the position of the baby within your pelvis. The fluid has a distinctive smell which helps to distinguish it from urine and you may notice an increase in the flow at the time of Braxton Hicks or true contractions. The membranes often go while in bed, which is why women are advised to sleep with polythene sheeting under the sheet, although this can make you unpleasantly sticky.

Labour usually starts within some hours of the membranes going. If you know the baby's head is engaged in the pelvis, you need only put on a pad or waterproof-backed nappy to soak up the fluid and carry on quietly as normal.

Contractions can start almost immediately or may take as long as several days to get going. Conventionally obstetricians like babies to be delivered within 24 hours of spontaneous rupture of membranes, and will want to induce you if labour is not well under way by then (see p. 98). This is because there can be an increased risk of infection to you or the baby from bacteria travelling up the vagina. Some will give you longer providing you take antibiotics. Some midwives take a more relaxed view and will leave it as long as six days before considering induction. If you do not want to be induced, try taking eight garlic perles and 1 g vitamin C several times a day to combat infection, and be scrupulous about hygiene. This means showering instead of bathing, using loo paper with care so that you wipe from front to back, and not introducing anything into the vagina so that you have no vaginal examinations, or sex. Try any of the methods of self-induction that do not involve contact with the vagina (see pp. 100–1). If your temperature is raised you may well have an infection which must be treated.

There are two situations where you need to take immediate action following ruptured membranes. One is if you know the baby's head is high (i.e. not well into the pelvis) or if you are not sure if it is engaged. The other is if the amniotic fluid that drains away is stained with meconium — the greenish-black contents of the baby's bowel. It might be any shade from green through brown to black. Fresh meconium, which might have been passed as a result of the baby being currently in distress, is green. It causes concern when it is thick as there is a risk of it clogging the baby's lungs if it is inhaled.

The risk with membranes rupturing while the head is still high is that there is a very slight chance that the umbilical cord might precede the baby's head into the birth canal. As contractions push the head downwards the cord can become pinched between the baby's head and the pelvis, cutting off the baby's blood supply. This only happens in 1 out of 400 deliveries and it is much more likely to happen when the membranes are ruptured artificially.

In both these cases you should call the midwife immediately or ring your doctor or hospital. If you know the head to be high, try and lie flat until you have been examined. If the cord is definitely protruding, call an ambulance straight away and lie face down with your knees on the ground and your bottom high in the air. Do not touch the cord except to push it carefully back into your vagina.

Change in cervix
This provides the most convincing evidence that labour

has started. If you are accustomed to feeling your cervix regularly you will be in a good position to notice the way it changes towards the end of pregnancy. A 'ripe' cervix, that is one which is ready for labour, feels soft and malleable, more like your lips to touch than your nose. It will have become softer, shorter and thinner and you may be able to get your finger in easily.

If you think you are in labour you can make sure by feeling your cervix. You MUST wash your hand thoroughly first (see p. 28). If your cervix is high or you can't reach it, you are unlikely to be in labour because the cervix descends and becomes easier to reach as it dilates. At this point, if it is accessible, it will feel as if the edges are frayed. It may feel wobbly and you might be able to get two fingers inside.

When you are definitely in labour, the baby's head moves down, and you will feel the cervix lower in your vagina. There will be nothing left of the canal of the cervix, it will have been taken up into the body of the uterus so that all that remains is the tissue stretched over the head, with the os or opening gradually getting wider. At this stage it may feel like something slimy over a grapefruit. It may be stretched taut so that you are unable to get your fingers inside it, or you may feel the plastic-like membranes with the amniotic fluid behind them. The hole left by the dilating cervix is completely round, and once it is fully dilated (10 cm), there is no rim of cervix left at all.

The chief advantage in doing your own vaginal examination would be to make sure you are in established labour (usually held to be 3–4 cm dilated) before taking your next step. There can be an interval of quite some hours between the start of contractions and reaching this stage, especially if it is your first baby.

Contractions

Many, but not all, women are aware of contractions of the uterus from about 20 weeks of pregnancy onwards. In fact the uterus is contracting at intervals throughout our lives. You may experience these contractions, known as

Braxton-Hicks, as occasions where the uterus seems to swell and become hard and tight. It lasts for about a minute and can make walking difficult. They tend to occur more often if you are exercising or if you have been sitting still for a long time.

As you get towards the end of pregnancy, these contractions can occur more frequently, last longer, and start to become uncomfortable. At this stage they may be starting to prepare you for labour by taking up your cervix. It can happen quite often that you get a spell of harder contractions with shorter intervals between them, which then fade away just at the point where you become convinced it is labour. If this happens during the night it can be helpful to have a hot drink together with a couple of paracetamol, or perhaps an alcoholic drink. This will not stop true labour, but will let you get a night's sleep if it is not.

Labour contractions become more frequent, last longer and are stronger. They may start by feeling like period pains or give you backache, or radiate down your thighs. The classic pattern is for them to start at half-hourly intervals, then gradually to come at intervals of 20 minutes, 15 and so on, until they are lasting up to two minutes with as little as a one minute interval between them. Of course not everyone fits this pattern, some may have contractions at five minute intervals until the end or they may last the same length of time or the contractions may come at irregular intervals.

WHEN TO GO INTO HOSPITAL

If you are going into hospital to have your baby, you will want to know when to go. This will obviously depend on circumstances such as how far from the hospital you live and whether you are likely to get caught up in rush-hour traffic, whether you have other children to be cared for and so on. However you might think it is time to go if:

- you are in labour before 36 weeks

- you are bleeding, even a heavy show
- you are in labour and your previous births were very quick (see also p. 110), although this is a good indication for home birth
- your membranes have ruptured, with a high head or the amniotic fluid is coloured (see p. 86)
- you are more than 5 cm dilated
- if you feel you cannot cope or are very frightened
- if contractions are every 5 minutes or more often and last longer than a minute, providing that you also feel that you need to go now.

It is obviously very difficult to gauge how strong the contractions are if this is your first labour and the risk is that you will go in too early, thus laying yourself open to the risks of intervention. It is best to hang on until you feel you absolutely cannot manage at home any longer. Try not to err on the safe side, and if you find that you are only slightly dilated when you get to the hospital, go home again.

LABOUR — WHAT HAPPENS

Labour itself consists of uterine contractions which initially alter the shape of the uterus so that from being a bag with a neck hanging down into the vagina, it becomes one unit, forming the birth canal. The contractions then change from those which pull the cervix upward, to being expulsive in nature so that the top of the uterus exerts pressure downward forcing the baby out through the vagina. This simple explanation belies what can be a process which may take many hours, be extremely painful and totally exhausting. It tends to go much more smoothly if you are happy in your surroundings, feel supported and are confident that you are in good hands. It can be more difficult if you are frightened, miserable, unhappy and do not feel at home in your situation or with those who are with you.

The first stage

The first stage of labour can take any time from days to minutes, although it is wise to allow 24 hours. In the early phase it can be very exciting as it is exhilarating to think you are finally about to get on with the event you have been awaiting for so long. At first you can get on with things normally, and you are able to talk through contractions. It is best to play down the drama at this point and save your 'breathing' until later. If it is night-time, find something to do which will take your mind off labour as everything appears to be more intense at night. Concentrating on something else can be very useful at this stage.

As the contractions get stronger you will find that you have to devote more attention to them and that you become less interested in what is going on around you. It may help to breathe through the contractions, using a simple technique of breathing in through the nose and out through the mouth *slowly*, concentrating on the outward breath, and deliberately relaxing your body. It also helps to keep mobile and remain in an upright position, perhaps rotating your hips like a belly dancer. By now you may feel that labour is a serious business, and you may be surprised by how painful the contractions are becoming, although you will probably feel fine in between.

Towards the end of the first stage of labour, say when the cervix is between 7–10 cm dilated, some women experience a phase known as transition. This is a combination of a physical and mental state where your legs might tremble, you may get cramp in them or your bottom, you may vomit or feel that you need to push before you are fully dilated. Mentally it can be a confusing time when you may feel that you can't cope any more, that the whole thing is a bad idea, and that you will give it up for the time being and resume later. You can be very irritable, swearing at everyone, want to go home even if you are already there. It can be a low point, where you feel as if you have used up all your energy and you are in despair.

The second stage

Transition can last from minutes to a couple of hours and some people never experience it. It ends when your cervix is fully dilated, which may coincide with your feeling the urge to push. This sensation which is initially felt at the height of a contraction, can be so overwhelming that you can do nothing but go with it. If you do not feel it, your body may be in a resting phase which can last up to half an hour. It is a mistake to start pushing before your body is ready.

Pushing should come naturally if you have had a drug-free labour and are in an upright position. However this does not mean that it will not be hard work — it can require every ounce of effort that you have got. It can help to make several short efforts with each contraction, deliberately relaxing your pelvic floor and pushing down with your diaphragm. It helps to visualise the baby coming down and round the curve of the birth canal. It can be a long process when the baby seems to move five steps forward and four back.

A squatting position, or supported squat, can be a good position for delivery, because that way there is no pressure on your coccyx which can impede progress and gravity assists the downward movement. The all-fours position can help to control a rapid delivery and is a good position during labour if the baby is posterior (has its back against your back with its limbs facing out), when it can assist the baby to turn so that it is presenting more favourably.

Some people find the second stage of labour from full dilatation to the birth, very painful and others welcome the opportunity to do something positive after a long period of allowing the body to do most of the work. Quite a few women find the moment of crowning when the baby's head comes through the stretched perineum as being like splitting, burning or bursting. Your midwife may tell you to pant rather than push at this point; if you can, you have a better chance of not tearing. You can guard your perineum with your hands — this may also help if you have difficulty in grasping exactly in which direction to push.

In the majority of births the baby's head will emerge facing towards your anus and then rotate so that it faces your thigh. The upper shoulder is helped to slide underneath the pubic arch, followed by the lower shoulder and then the rest of the body slithers out.

When you first see your baby it may look blue-purple until it takes its first breath when it rapidly turns pink. It can be quite slippery and messy, and may be covered in vernix, the white waterproof cream that protects its skin while in the amniotic fluid. It may look waterlogged or streaked with blood and mucus and have a thick blue and white cord coming from its navel. The genitals of either sex can be astonishingly prominent. The baby's head may have been moulded during birth so that its shape looks most unnatural and it will be swollen around its eyes. Breast feeding is most likely to succeed if it is put to your breast straightaway.

The third stage

The final stage of labour may be overlooked by you in the excitement of meeting your baby at last. The emotion felt at this time and stimulation of the baby's sucking results in the production of oxytocin from the pituitary gland into the blood-stream. This has an effect on the uterus which then contracts and becomes smaller so that the placenta is forced to peel away. Further contractions should ensure that it is delivered soon after the baby. It resembles a large piece of liver.

PAIN RELIEF IN LABOUR — THE OPTIONS

Nearly everyone finds labour very painful and feels at some point that they would like something to relieve the pain.

Orthodox methods of pain relief

The pharmacological methods available on the NHS are Entonox, pethidine or Meptid, and epidural anaesthesia. All have some disadvantages and are only available in hospital or from a community midwife.

Entonox is the least intrusive. It is a mixture of nitrous oxide and oxygen which is inhaled through a mask or mouthpiece. It works best if you take several deep breaths through it at the start of a contraction, so that the gas is effective when you reach the peak. It can make you feel as if you have had a couple of gins, and it is useful in taking the edge off the pain. You cannot take too much because your hand drops from the mask when you have had enough. The gas is rapidly eliminated from your body and the oxygen benefits the baby. The disadvantages are that you have to stay close to the cylinder and it makes some women feel sick.

Pethidine and Meptid are anti-spasmodic drugs given by intra-muscular injection. They have a place as relaxants but they also have several disadvantages. Pethidine, for instance, is not especially good at relieving pain and can make the baby floppy at birth if it is given between three hours and half an hour before the birth; it also takes at least 10 minutes to work and it can make you feel sick or drowsy; some women even have hallucinations when they use it. Meptid relieves the pain but does not have the same relaxant effect.

If the baby is born with breathing difficulties or you feel that the injection has been a mistake, there is an antidote, Narcan, which can be given, either to the baby or you.

The advantage of pethidine is that it can help if you feel that tension is slowing the progress of the labour. Ask for a small dose of 50–70 mg, though make sure that you are examined beforehand, because if you are 7 cm or more dilated it might not be worth it.

Epidural anaesthesia involves injecting an anaesthetic agent into the epidural space around your spinal cord. If it is well placed, it takes away all sensation of pain from the uterus while leaving some feeling in your legs. It is good in long or difficult labours, when a caesarean section is necessary and for lowering raised blood pressure.

The disadvantage is that it can slow down labour, that forceps are needed more often with an epidural because you can lose the urge to push, and it may prevent the muscles of the perineum from rotating the baby's head at birth. You also have to have a drip up and be under continuous monitoring. An epidural means that you are restricted to the bed and that it will be difficult to adopt an upright position for delivery.

An epidural has to be administered by a specially trained anaesthetist, with you sitting or lying on the bed with your knees up and your back curved as much as possible. It is important to lie still while the anaesthetist is working which can be difficult when you are having contractions. First a local anaesthetic is administered to numb the area round the spine and then a hollow needle is inserted into your spine. Once it is in the right place, a fine catheter is threaded through the needle, and the needle is then removed. The tube is taped up your back to your shoulder and the anaethetising agent is injected through the filter at the top of the tube. It takes about 20 minutes to work and you will be rolled from side to side to ensure the drug is evenly distributed. Sometimes the epidural fails to work or only works down one side. There is a small risk that the dura may be punctured which will cause a severe headache and means that you will have to be nursed on your back for several days. There is also a very remote risk of paralysis.

Alternative pain relief

There are alternative ways of relieving the pain of childbirth. Few can remove the pain completely, but they are free from side effects to you and your baby. All of them are more effective if you have plenty of support and encouragement. One study concluded that good support is equal to a full dose of pethidine in its ability to reduce the appreciation of pain. Some simple measures that might help include using a hot water bottle on your back or front, and massage. Try taking six tablets of Dolomite at the start of labour in order to provide a boost of calcium to compensate for the large amounts required by the contracting muscles. If preferred effervescent calcium can be taken in water, 1 g every 3 hours.

Herbal remedies
Coriander is recommended by Juliette de Bairacli Levy in her book *The Illustrated Herbal Handbook*. She suggests taking three or four sprays of leaves eaten raw as a salad herb, or half a teaspoon of the seeds, mixed with honey and eaten raw, or making a tea from the seeds. Raspberry leaf tea can be drunk freely throughout labour, or it can be taken as previously prepared ice cubes. Poppyhead tea can also help with pain-relief — take six fresh or dried poppyheads in ½ pint (300 ml) of water. Susun Weed, American herbalist, author of *Wise Women Herbal for the Childbearing Years*, recommends three drops of skullcap and 25 drops of St John's wort tinctures taken every hour if needed.

Aromatherapy
Use clary sage in the massage oil.

Acupuncture
If you can have an acupuncturist with you in labour he or she can relieve pain and speed up the labour if necessary. They can also stop any nausea. It takes about 10 minutes to work and does not remove pain completely, but reduces it to a bearable level. TNS has a similar effect.

Transcutaneous Nerve Stimulation (TNS)
This method of pain relief is available in some hospitals and can also be hired. It is a small battery-operated device which delivers a minute charge of electricity to the nerves that supply the uterus at the point where they go into the spine. It works by stimulating endorphins — the body's natural opiates — and by helping to prevent the message of pain from getting to the brain. Four electrodes covered in conductive gel are taped to your back and connected to the TNS machine by means of a lead. A push button handset allows you to alter the mode of operation between

the on-off mode which gives an intermittent pulse which is used between contractions and a continuous mode used during contractions. A dial allows you to increase the impulse.

It is best used from early labour and takes about 20 minutes to work. The sensation is a bit like pins and needles. Most women find it helpful and some need no other pain relief. It works well in combination with Entonox.

The disadvantage is that it cannot be used with a bath or shower and it may interfere with a fetal scalp monitor. If you intend to use a hospital machine you either have to go in early in order to use it or risk putting it on later than would otherwise be ideal.

An obstetric TNS machine is available for hire for four weeks from £20.00 from Neen Pain Management Systems (see p. 184).

Massage
Massage can be wonderful for relieving pain and tension. It is effective during pregnancy when it can alleviate the aches that are an inevitable part of carrying a baby, and it can be enormously helpful in labour. Use talcum powder or a vegetable oil to which a few drops of an essential oil have been added to lubricate the skin. Some suggested techniques are:

- stroking gently but firmly from the shoulder to the tips of the fingers
- placing your hands on the shoulders and massaging the neck and shoulders with your thumbs
- firm stroking of the inside or outside of the thighs
- pushing the heel of your hand hard against the base of the spine and rubbing in a circular motion so that the skin moves over the bone and there is no friction between the skin and the hand — this is very good for backache
- supporting the woman's head while she is leaning forward so that she can rest its whole weight in your

hand — you need to be well-braced to do this
- stroking gently up from the forehead into the hairline
- press your thumbs firmly into the centre of the buttocks to relieve backache
- either just hold the feet firmly when pain is making her twist them together, or support a foot with one hand and stroke the sole firmly with the heel of your other hand
- apply deep pressure with your thumbs in a line down the centre of the sole to the heel

Massage needs to be done in a smooth, rhythmic sequence. However, bear in mind that women sometimes cannot bear to be touched while they are in labour or find that some types of massage which were previously enjoyed are unhelpful, so you need to be sensitive to her changing needs.

Homeopathic remedies
See remedies for labour, chapter 9.

You should take each contraction as it comes and know that you are coping if you cope with that one. It is not a good idea to anticipate and think that you cannot stand another few hours of labouring like that because childbirth is entirely unpredictable and even experienced midwives can be wrong in their predictions of how long your labour will last. Basing your decisions on estimates can mean that you choose forms of pain relief that you would prefer not to use. You do however need to keep an open mind, as labour can be far more painful than you anticipate.

9.
WHEN LABOUR IS NOT STRAIGHTFORWARD

INDUCTION

Labour is sometimes induced for sound medical reasons, such as if the mother's blood pressure is high and continuing to rise, or the baby is hardly moving or there is proven growth retardation. However induction is often pressed because the consultant has a policy of inducing everyone who is a certain number of days overdue; this can even be on the due date in certain cases or it might be as long as two weeks. Some consultants do not induce without a medical indication and surveys are beginning to show that mothers and babies do better without this intervention. Labour goes most smoothly when it is spontaneous.

There will always be a reason given for your induction, but the fact that there is no consensus on the risks of prolonged labour, together with the fact that the stage where you are considered dangerously overdue will depend on where you are having the baby, means that you can resist the offer if you want. You may like to have the baby's heartbeat monitored on a cardiotocograph, a belt monitor which will make a trace of its heart readings and your contractions if any. Regular monitoring for periods of half an hour will show how well the baby is withstanding the rigours of life in utero.

Medical induction can consist of the following measures:

- Sweep of membranes — this is where a midwife or

doctor inserts a finger into your cervix and sweeps it around the top so that the lower membranes become detached. This often initiates labour, but it can only be done if your cervix is already ripe.

- Prostin pessary — this is a pessary containing prostaglandins which is given in hospital to ripen the cervix with the aim of starting labour. It is often given the night before a full induction and can send you into spontaneous labour.

- Artificial rupture of the membranes — membranes are ruptured by means of an amnihook which looks like a plastic crochet hook and is inserted through the cervix to snag the membranes so that the amniotic fluid is lost. This often starts labour and is also used to accelerate a labour which has started spontaneously. The disadvantage, apart from the fact that it is done in hospital, is that it can be very painful if the cervix is not ripe, that it might put you suddenly into very strong labour and that most consultants consider that they are committed by delivering you within 24 hours, even if necessary by caesarean section, because of the risk that infection has been introduced to the baby by the amniotomy.

- Syntocinon drip — this is synthetic oxytocin administered through a drip in the arm. This may be used if other methods have failed or it may be put up at the same time as the membranes are ruptured. It usually starts contractions, the strength of which can be controlled by altering the amount of Syntocinon. The disadvantages are that artificially stimulated contractions can be a lot harder to cope with than natural ones so that you may need more pain relief than you otherwise would, and if you have an epidural you are more likely to need forceps. You will be asked to accept continuous monitoring because there is a risk of over-stimulation of the uterus. There is a greater risk of your baby becoming jaundiced or requiring special care. If Syntocinon fails you will be delivered by caesarean section.

Alternatives to induction

These alternative methods for triggering of an overdue
labour are not fool-proof, but have a certain amount of
success and are well worth trying if you think that you are
going to have to agree to a medical induction.

- Sex — semen contains prostaglandin so can work in
  the same way as the Prostin pessary, although the
  prostaglandin is less concentrated in semen. Frequent
  sex, followed by lying on your back with a pillow under
  your bottom for at least half an hour can therefore
  sometimes start labour.
- Nipple stimulation — twiddling your nipples for 15
  minutes or more at a time stimulates the release of
  oxytocin and thus labour.
- Curry — this is a purgative working on the same
  principle as castor oil, but rather more palatable. Have
  as hot a curry as you can stand.
- Castor oil — take a third of a tumbler mixed well with
  liver salts or orange juice. Unfortunately it is
  unpleasant to take and is followed by violent
  diarrhoea. However it can start labour if you are on the
  brink and it clears the bowel so that you will not need
  a suppository, but if it works you may start labour
  feeling rather weak.
- Sweep of membranes (see p. 98) — you can try
  stretching your cervix manually yourself.
- Homeopathic remedy — take Caulophyllum 30 every
  half an hour until contractions start.
- Cranial osteopathy — a cranial osteopath can get
  labour started by working via your pituitary gland,
  although it takes a couple of days to take effect.
- Herbal remedies — goldenseal is an oxytocic herb.
  Try taking 2.5 ml of the tincture every hour until
  contractions are regular. It is extremely bitter, so have
  a sweet ready to suck after taking it. Labour tincture
  is a recipe from *The Wise Woman Herbal for the
  Childbearing Year* by Susun Weed. It might be wise
  make up this herbal remedy at least six weeks before

you are due if you think you are at risk of induction.
You will need:

½ oz (15 g) dried black cohosh root
½ oz (15 g) dried blue cohosh root
¼ oz (10 g) dried ginger
¼ oz (10 g) dried beth root
11 fl oz (325 ml) vodka

Put the dried herbs in a large, opaque jar and add the
vodka. Label the jar clearly and cap it. Allow the mixture
to steep for at least six weeks. When you want to decant it,
put it into a juice extractor or pour into a muslin cloth and
squeeze out as much liquid as you can. Store in a brown,
glass container in a cool dark place. When the tincture is
required, take 10 drops under the tongue every hour until
contractions are regular. Castor oil rubbed into the
abdomen and covered with a warm towel may also help
trigger off labour if the cervix is ripe.

EPISIOTOMY

An episiotomy is a cut made into your perineum (the skin
between the vagina and the anus) in order to enlarge the
outlet for the baby. It is one of the aspects of childbirth
that is most dreaded and disliked. It is done when the
baby's head is stretching the perineum, by infusing the
area with local anaesthetic and then cutting it with very
sharp scissors. The cut is made from the vagina outwards
and backwards, slanting away from the rectum. It may be
done without an anaesthetic in an emergency because the
perineum is numbed naturally by the stretching.

Some of the reasons for doing an episiotomy include:
fetal distress, having a rigid perineum which is holding the
baby in, a forceps delivery for whatever reason, it looks as
if you might tear, all first-time mothers in this hospital
have episiotomies and all subsequent mothers who have
had episiotomy previously must have a repeat. Some
midwives are not used to doing deliveries without them.

Clearly some reasons have more validity than others,

and you are dependent to some extent on the skill of your attendants. Some midwives take a particular pride in delivering so that a cut or tear is avoided. A tear may be preferred to a cut if damage is inevitable because it will follow the natural stress line, instead of cutting through muscle, and because it heals better and more comfortably. The edges, being irregular, knit together like a jigsaw, although an episiotomy having straight edges, is easier to suture. Moreover you have the slight satisfaction of knowing that it has not been done routinely. Make sure your attendants know if you would prefer to tear; you are not always asked before an episiotomy is done. Some midwives feel that tears heal best with few or no stitches. The bruising will be minimised, the blood loss less and there will be fewer problems with infection and healing if you take Arnica 200 just before and just after delivery.

Obviously prevention is better than cure and there are a number of ways of avoiding the problem. The first is the long-term measure of perineal massage (see p. 39) and the second is by taking care at the time of birth. This can be done by applying a flannel wrung out in hot water to the perineum to soften the tissues. Massaging with oil in the second stage can also help the baby to slide out without trauma. When the baby's head crowns you need to control your breathing so that you stop pushing and allow the head to slip out. Your midwife may ask you to pant, and it is vital to do this although you may well feel that you are past caring. The more slowly the head emerges the greater the opportunity for the perineum to stretch and accommodate it. You can help by reaching down to feel your baby's head and helping to guide it out.

The position that you deliver in can make a difference to your chances of tearing — upright, squatting or all-fours are best, all-fours probably providing the best opportunity for control. Lying flat or semi-sitting positions are more likely to result in damage.

If you do have stitches they may not necessarily bother you, but they can cause enormous pain and discomfort, making the post-partum period misery. At its worst, sitting can be so painful that it is impossible to find a comfortable position in which to feed and some women are forced to feed standing up.

The pain does go in the end and your perineum heals over, although it can be a deterrent to sex for quite a while. Making love with the pressure off the scar and using KY jelly may help, but if your scar is not comfortable by the time of your post-natal check, make sure that your doctor appreciates the fact. Occasionally poor stitching needs re-doing. Make sure that you get a midwife or experienced doctor to suture you, and beware — medical students first learn to suture on perineums!

Practical tips include: applying ice packs or ice in tough plastic bags or bags of frozen peas to the area, throwing a handful of salt into your bath as an antiseptic, taking the pressure off by sitting on an inflatable rubber ring (available from chemists), sitting in a basin of hot and cold water alternately, keeping stitches dry by using your hairdryer on them. Ultrasound treatment can increase the inflammatory phase and stimulate the healing process.

Herbal remedies
Bathe the wound with a few drops of calendula tincture in warm water or use the solution in a spray.

You can also make a paste with slippery elm bark and water, olive oil, vitamin E oil and comfrey powder if you have it. Spread it onto muslin and hold it in place with a pad. Change it every time you go to the loo. Arnica cream, not ointment, around the stitch line will help ease bruising. Calendula or hypercal cream will assist healing. Once the wound has healed, try massaging the scar with vitamin E or comfrey oil.

Homeopathic remedies
Take Arnica 200, this will need to be followed by Calendula for some days. If the episiotomy was done against your wishes, take staphysagria.

FORCEPS DELIVERY

Forceps are needed to help a baby out in around 5 per cent of births, although they may be used far more frequently. They can be needed in cases of fetal distress, maternal exhaustion, and when the baby's head is well down into the pelvis but progress has halted, often when an epidural is in use. They are occasionally used for premature babies, breech births and to deliver babies born by caesarean section.

If forceps are suggested, it is likely to be at a point where you may be at your lowest, having been pushing for some time and you may feel that you do not care what is done to you. It is, however, worth making a superhuman effort to avoid forceps. This means getting into a squatting position — even if you have had an epidural anaesthetic and cannot feel your legs. Ask those around you to support you, and it may help to hold on to the end of the bed.

Some hospitals have policies about the length of time that you are allowed in the second stage before they use forceps. This may be as little as an hour for a first baby and half an hour for a second. You should be allowed as long as it takes, provided you and the baby are coping. It helps to wait until the urge to push is overwhelming; remember there may be a resting phase of as much as half an hour between full dilatation and feeling the need to push. Pushing with a high head when you do not want to makes forceps more likely.

A forceps delivery is done by a doctor, while you lie flat on your back on the delivery bed. Your legs are placed in stirrups on either side and your perineum is injected with local anaesthetic, and an episiotomy performed. Once the anaesthetic takes effect, both blades of the forceps are inserted into your vagina separately. They consist of a hollow metal guard which curves round the baby's head and a shaft which is angled to go round the curve of the birth canal.

Once the blades are in position, they are locked together

so that the head cannot be crushed. With each contraction the doctor pulls and you push; sometimes it requires an astonishing amount of effort. Once the head is out, you push your baby's body out yourself. The resulting depression of the temporal bones may mean that the baby is slow to start to breathe.

Delivery by forceps can give you quite severe bruising and a very sore perineum. You will probably want to try the remedies for episiotomy (see p. 103) and take Arnica at the time followed by Calendula for several days, together with Bellis Perennis for soft tissue injury and Staphysagria for emotions and shock.

A baby delivered by forceps would benefit from treatment from a cranial osteopath when it is 14 days old. It can also be helped with the flower remedies, Star of Bethlehem for trauma and walnut to help it adjust to change. Mix as recommended on p. 8 and drop into the mouth. The homeopathic remedies are Arnica, and if after that the baby is fractious and twitchy, it should be given Kali Phos 6x.

FAILURE OF LABOUR TO PROGRESS OR SLOW LABOUR

This is when you start labour and are having regular, painful contractions but the cervix fails to dilate. It may not dilate at all or it may get to some stage below full dilatation (10 cm) and then stop. The causes can include not being able to let go because you are frightened or the atmosphere is inhibiting, progress being halted by epidural anaesthesia, and occasionally disproportion when your pelvis is not big enough to take this particular baby.

If you feel inhibited by the atmosphere or by particular birth attendants, you or your partner will have to have the courage to alter the situation. It is not surprising that many labours slow down or stop as soon as couples reach hospital, because you can feel yourself to be on alien territory there, uncertain about what is going on and amongst people you do not know. The same thing can happen when someone you feel is not sympathetic comes to your home when you are in labour. If progress has stopped, ask everyone to leave you alone for at least 15 minutes, if necessary leave the hospital and go home. This can be just as effective and a lot more pleasant than having a Syntocinon drip put up, the orthodox remedy in this case. It might help to have a bath. Tell yourself 'open' and visualise your cervix opening up. Make sure you keep altering your position and that you are being massaged. Nipple rolling or stimulation stimulates oxytocin and can encourage labour too.

You have a right to be allocated a different midwife if you are not getting on well with the one you have — ask the sister in charge, or ring the supervisor of the community midwives and see if she could send someone else. The chances are that if you are not seeing eye to eye, she will be glad of a change too.

If an epidural seems to have stopped progress you will have to allow it to wear off and then not have it renewed, which may be difficult to accept. Pethidine is useful in this instance, it can often relax you enough for the cervix to dilate. The usual approach in hospital is to further stimulate contractions by means of a Syntocinon drip, and, if that fails, to deliver the baby by caesarean section.

Alternative remedies

These include having a glass of wine or beer, applying pressure from your nail or a matchstick to bladder 67 — the point beside the nail of your little toe — or using reflexology to encourage a sluggish labour by holding a strong comb in each hand during a contraction and gripping them tightly so that they press on the mid-finger tips and the balls of the hands. It may also help to have someone apply firm pressure to the centre of the balls of your feet.

Herbal remedies

You could try taking $\frac{1}{4}$–$\frac{1}{2}$ teaspoonful of bethroot tincture. Or 10–20 drops of blue and black cohosh roots —

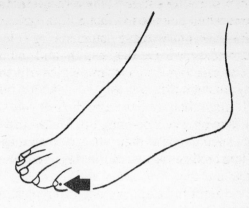

Acupressure point to stimulate contractions

Apply pressure to the point beside your little toenail with a matchstick
or your nail.

these two should be combined and not used singly. If you
have the labour tincture ready made (see p. 101), take 10
drops under the tongue at half-hour intervals.

Homeopathic remedies

If the contractions are changeable, dilation is slow and you
are tearful, take Pulsatilla. If the contractions are relaxed,
you are getting 'false pains', tiring, or slowing down, take
Gelsemium.

Veronica was expecting her second baby. Her previous
child had been a forceps delivery after a long labour and
it had been suggested that her pelvis was inadequate.
Her waters went at 4.00 pm and she went to hospital at
midnight. By 2.00 am labour was established but at
3.00 contractions stopped. By 4.00 there were still no
contractions and she was threatened with a drip. By
this time Veronica was anxious but not frightened. The
anxiety was treated with Aconite. She was also given
Caulophyllum 6 every fifteen minutes. By 4.45 strong
contractions were under way and at 6.30 the baby was

born without problems. By 7.30 the placenta had not
been delivered Syntometrine was not given) and the
hospital staff were becoming anxious. Caulophyllum
200 was given as a single dose and the placenta arrived
ten minutes later.

Aromatherapy
A bath with a few drops of clary sage, being a euphoric,
or massage with clary sage oil in the base, will also help
labour along.

EXHAUSTION IN LABOUR
Labour can be extremely tiring, which is why it is an
advantage to be as fit as possible at the start. It is
exhausting to be intermittently in severe pain, and
even if you are totally relaxed throughout, your body is
still using up large amounts of energy which can mean
that long before the end you can feel that you have
had enough and that you would be happy to call it
a day. As this option is unlikely to be open to you,
you need to consider the others. The best way to conserve
energy is to relax through contractions and, if this
proves impossible, to rest completely between them.
Relaxation techniques are taught in most ante-natal
classes.

Exhaustion is frequently exacerbated by a policy of not
feeding a woman in labour. This is because it is thought to
be safer in the event of your needing a general anaesthetic,
because you are at risk of suffocating if you inhale vomit.
However it is now known that it is more dangerous to
inhale the acid that accumulates in the stomach if you are
not allowed to eat than to inhale partially-digested food,
which does not burn the lungs. It is most unlikely that this
will happen and it seems probable that starving labouring
women does more harm in leaving them exhausted so that
they need more intervention.

In many cases the digestion tends to shut down during

labour, so that any food you do have should be light and
easily digested. If your system cannot cope with what you
have eaten, it will send it back. One remedy is to take
fructose — fruit sugar — in drinks or powdered. This is
preferable to glucose because it provides a sustained
release of energy instead of an initial peak followed by a
trough. Fructose is available from health food shops.

Pethidine can help you get some sleep if you are
completely exhausted, although you may find you wake
up in the middle of a contraction, unprepared for it and
unable to cope.

It is at this point that you may agree to procedures that
beforehand you felt certain that you did not want.
Obviously you should be free to change your mind as the
situation demands, but it can be useful for a partner to be
aware of the possible state of mind that exhaustion brings
and to be very sympathetic and encouraging. You can
sometimes regret giving in, although it is hard afterwards
to remember just how little strength you may have felt
you had.

Herbal remedies
Herbal remedies include taking either ginger or wild
ginger, either as 15–20 drops in water or as 2–5 drops
under the tongue. Drinking raspberry leaf tea throughout
the labour can speed it up. The other herb which might
help is pure ginseng; take 2–4 capsules every 4 hours.

Bach flower remedies
Take Rescue Remedy frequently as labour progresses.
You might also add olive and oak flower remedies.

Homeopathic remedies
For ineffectual contractions which are exhausting and not
getting anywhere, take Caulophyllum. For exhausting
contractions and labour that is going on too long, take Kali
Phos and Rescue Remedy. These can be taken all the way
through if necessary. For doubling up and shivering in the
first stage, take Cimicifuga. For transition — unbearable

pains, you are irritable or capricious, and feel worse with warmth, take Chamomilla. Pains made much worse by the slightest movement or touch, and you want to go home, take Bryonia. In the second stage when the head appears with each contraction, only to disappear again, take Silica. For exhaustion, take Kali Phos.

Stephanie was having her first baby at home. Labour progressed normally for eight hours. Suddenly the pains became intolerable, nothing was right, she wanted rubbing, then she didn't, all positions were uncomfortable — in short she was in transition. She was given Chamomilla 6 with each contraction. An hour later she started to push, was having strong contractions and was fully dilated. An hour later she was still pushing and not feeling too tired. Another hour passed and she was still pushing and getting tired in the squatting position, the midwives were starting to think about 'doing something'. The baby's heart was fine. Arnica 200 was given as a single dose. Half an hour later the baby's head appeared with each push, only to disappear again. She took a single dose of Silica 200 and the baby was born 15 minutes later. The placenta came away 45 minutes later. Stephanie was very bruised from pushing so long and so took Arnica 200 immediately after the birth and another dose later.

PRECIPITATE (TOO FAST) LABOUR

It can happen that you go into labour very rapidly. This is much more likely to occur if this is not your first baby. There are effective delaying tactics, but the best remedy is for you to feel confident that you can deliver the baby yourself. If labour proceeds that rapidly, nature is working at its best and there is very rarely any problem with either mother and baby.

If you feel that your baby is arriving suddenly (overwhelming desire to push, great sensation of

something like a grapefruit in the rectum), ring a
midwife or an ambulance. You can delay the birth by
adopting the knee-chest position, that is with your bottom
high in the air and your head on your crossed arms on the
floor. You can do this on the back seat of a car if you are
en route for the hospital. It is important to remember that
all that is necessary is to catch the baby and keep it warm
until you get help.

If you are delivering your own baby in an emergency:

- Find a towel or blanket to wrap the baby in — it is
  vital that the baby is kept warm.
- Find a soft spot on which to deliver, put a towel down
  if possible.
- When you feel the baby's head coming through your
  perineum, cup it with your hand.
- Once the head is out, feel for any loops of cord round
  the neck and bring them forward. The baby's head will
  probably emerge facing your anus and then rotate to
  face your thigh.
- Wipe the baby's eyes and mouth free of mucus with a
  clean hanky or your finger.
- Wait for the next contraction, and with it, guide the
  baby's head down so that its upper shoulder can slide
  underneath your pubic arch and, once it is free, guide
  the head upwards so that the lower shoulder can be
  freed and its body will follow.
- Wrap the baby up warmly as soon as possible and put
  it to the breast.
- The placenta will probably come away within half an
  hour, especially if you are upright and feeding the
  baby. If no help has arrived by the time the placenta
  has been delivered, wrap it separately from the baby
  and keep the two together. Do not cut or tie the cord.
- If you have not already done so, send for help. Take
  Rescue Remedy for shock! A baby that has been born
  very quickly may benefit from taking Arnica for the
  shock. If the baby shows signs of being fractious in the
  first few weeks of life, consider cranial osteopathy (see
  p. 9).

FAILURE OF BABY TO BREATHE

The seconds before the baby breathes can seem an age. If the baby is blue or purple at birth, it will definitely breathe within a minute or so. Occasionally, however, a baby is born in less good condition, in which case it may be white or grey in colour and not start to breathe spontaneously. If it is not breathing a minute after birth, it will be given oxygen from a mask held over its face. If that does not work, a tube will be put into its lungs to push air directly into them.

If the baby is born unexpectedly at home and fails to breathe, which is most unlikely, there are steps that you can take. Firstly, if possible call medical help. Make sure that you have hooked any mucus in the mouth out with your finger, or suck it out with a straw and tip the baby so that any remaining mucus can drain out of its mouth. Do not cut the cord, as the baby needs all the oxygen it can get from the placenta while the cord is pulsing. Stroke the baby's back and tell it why you want it here and flick the soles of its feet with your fingers. You can put Rescue Remedy into the baby's mouth and on the pulse points at wrist and temples. If all else fails do mouth-to-mouth resuscitation and heart massage if the heart beat is less than 60 beats a minute. Don't give up hope — babies can survive undamaged for 12 minutes without oxygen and may start breathing voluntarily.

POST-PARTUM HAEMORRHAGE

Heavy bleeding after the baby is born can be terrifying. Even a normal amount, considered to be 500 ml or less, seems like a lot. If the haemorrhage, which can either be a gush or a persistent trickle, starts shortly after the birth, your midwife will give you an intravenous injection of ergometrine. This has the effect of contracting your uterus and the site of the bleeding within 40 seconds. If you lose a lot of blood, you will require a blood transfusion. Occasionally a haemorrhage will occur in the two or three weeks following the birth. In this case ring your midwife immediately.

Alternative remedies
Put a piece of placenta in your mouth if it has been delivered, pinch your ankle hard at the point between your ankle bones, and sip half a cup of warm water in which a teaspoonful of cayenne has been dissolved.

Herbal remedies
Take 20 drops of blue cohosh or labour tincture, together with 50 drops of ground ivy tincture. Repeat after 2–5 minutes as necessary.

Homeopathic remedies
Haemorrhaging is unlikely to occur if you take Arnica and Kali Phos at birth. If it does occur, see the remedies given for miscarriage with reference to the type of bleeding (see pp. 46–7). For bright red bleeding, take Phosphorus. For bleeding accompanied by nausea, take Ipecac. If the bleeding is associated with faintness and dizziness which gets worse with the slightest movement, take Trillium.

CAESAREAN SECTION

This method of delivering babies is on the increase. The national average is above 10 per cent, with some hospitals having a rate of 25 per cent or more. It is an operation that can save lives and prevent brain damage, but its price can be high in physical, emotional and financial terms so that it should never be regarded as an easy option.

Elective caesarean section
There are various reasons why you might be booked for an elective caesarean section, that is one done on a pre-determined date. These include: *placenta praevia* — when the placenta blocks the cervix either totally or in part; very *high blood pressure* which cannot be controlled, as induced labour may deprive the baby of oxygen; a

previous caesarean section (although this in itself should not be an indication for a repeat caesarean unless the reason for the first one is recurring); a *contracted pelvis*, when your pelvis is permanently damaged by injury of disease; a *small pelvis* (although again this alone is not necessarily a good reason as the dimensions of the pelvis can expand by as much as 5 cm in labour and most women have the right-sized baby for their size; if you want to avoid a caesarean section for this reason, practise squatting, consult a cranial osteopath and take the remedies for easing delivery given on p. 106). If you suffer from *herpes*, a caesarean delivery will be performed if you have active sores because of the risk of passing the infection on to the baby (see p. 63 for remedies for herpes). Another indication for a caesarean section is *transverse ie*, when the baby lies across you and not vertically. Some consultants also perform caesarean sections for *breech* presentations (see p. 47).

Emergency caesarean section

If a caesarean section becomes necessary during the course of labour, see if it is possible to have the operation performed under epidural anaesthetic. This has two advantages: it is better physically — the baby gets less of the drug and you feel fitter afterwards — and it is better emotionally because you see your baby born and have no doubts about it being yours, and you can feed it almost straightaway.

The reasons for an emergency caesarean section include: *premature labour* — doctors sometimes prefer to deliver by caesarean section if premature labour cannot be stopped, although this is done less frequently as it is now realised that some stress helps the baby to adapt to being born; *placental abruption*, when the placenta starts to come away from the wall of the uterus before labour, leading to pain and bleeding; *cord prolapse* (see p. 86) when the cord descends first and is compressed as the baby comes down, cutting off blood supply; *fetal distress* if the baby becomes short of oxygen while still unborn, it is said to be in distress. The distress manifests itself as an alteration in the baby's heart-rate which either becomes very fast — above 160 beats per minute — or too slow, below 100 beats per minute. It is normal for the baby's heart-beat to slow at the same time as contractions, but less healthy for it to slow down once the contraction is over. Distress may also be shown by the baby discharging meconium into the amniotic fluid, although this does not definitely prove that something is wrong.

If your baby is showing signs of distress, you can help by moving on to all-fours and breathing oxygen from a mask. If the heart-beat drops suddenly and drastically, or gradually deteriorates before you are in the second stage of labour, a caesarean section will be done to reduce the risks to the baby. Other reasons for an emergency caesarean section are *failure to progress* (see pp. 105–8); *obstructed labour*, which is when the baby eventually presents abnormally, either by face, brow or shoulder in a position which cannot be altered or delivered vaginally; *failed induction; failed forceps* — if you are unlucky enough to need forceps and their use and squatting fails to deliver the baby, then it has to be born by caesarean section.

After the operation

Although recovery from the operation is relatively rapid, you will, nonetheless, be recovering from a major operation at the same time as starting a demanding career as the mother of a new baby, and it is important for everyone around you to appreciate that fact.

At first the post-operative pain will be controlled by drugs, but within a few days you will find that you can start to manage without them. A TNS electrode either side of the scar can provide drug-free pain relief. You will be encouraged to be up and about within a day or so, although you will still need help to get in and out of bed. It is difficult to stand upright at first because of the alarming but erroneous impression that your stomach is about to fall out through your stitches.

Pillows are invaluable for helping you maintain your position in bed and assisting you to balance the baby so that it is in a comfortable position for feeding and cuddling. It can be quite a shock to discover just how little you can do for yourself at first — you may need to hold on to the bedhead to pull yourself up to a sitting position, and you will certainly need help with turning in bed and feeding the baby.

You will be on a fluid diet at first, progressing quite rapidly to light food. Fruit cordials and soft fruit are very welcome in the early days. The third day after the operation is notorious for being the one in which you will be contorted with enormous amounts of wind. This can be helped by drinking peppermint water, available from the hospital. You can also get a flatus tube so that you make less of a racket. The homeopathic remedy Raphanus 30, available from pharmacies, is excellent for painful wind as a result of a caesarean section.

Although you may feel quite fit by the time you leave hospital, life is much harder when you get back home so that it is essential that you have lots of efficient help.

Homeopathic remedies

Take Arnica followed by Calendula for several days. If the operation was against your wishes take Staphysagria. Spray the wound with Calendula mother tincture, diluted 1:10. The baby should have Arnica after birth and Kali Phos if fractious or twitchy.

Babies delivered by caesarean section can also benefit from cranial osteopathy, because they need the rhythmic squeeze of contractions to initiate a healthy cranial rhythm.

Acupuncture

Treatment by acupuncture is useful to treat a scar that remains painful or does not heal well.

10.
AFTER BIRTH

How will you feel immediately after your baby is born?
You may feel either elated or exhausted, depending on the
circumstances. What you are unlikely to be able to do is
sleep, no matter how long is was since you last slept. After
an initial feed your baby is likely to settle to sleep leaving
you more awake than you have ever been, pondering over
and over again recent events. This period of wakefulness
seems to be essential for you to be able to make sense of
the monumental happenings and changes to your life that
have taken place.

At home this can be a family time, and you will be able
to eat and drink exactly what you want. In hospital, on the
other hand, food will be limited to what is available, and
you may well be ravenous. However try and ensure you
have some time together as a family, although this will
depend on the pressure on space in the delivery rooms.
Eventually, though, your companions will have to leave the
hospital and the two of you will be left alone.

Sooner or later you will become aware of the way your
body is feeling. Although it is a topic which is not much
discussed and something that you do not anticipate when
you are still concentrating on how labour will go, the
reality of the early post-partum period can be quite a
shock. For months, you and the baby have been one large,
perhaps uncomfortable, but self-contained unit and then
quite suddenly you are separate. You and the baby are
likely to feel the difference — you seem to be leaking from
every orifice, you will be sweating a lot, starting to leak
milk, weeing copiously, and, surprisingly after nine or so
bleed-free months, bleeding heavily. You may scarcely
recollect what a sanitary pad is, when you find that
suddenly you are soaking the mega-maternity versions at
an alarming rate.

The baby too is quite a different proposition. Whether you find your baby adorable or you are still coming to terms with his or her existence — and you may well not fall instantly in love with your infant — he or she will soon make it clear that they need attention too. Babies are often sleepy for the first day or two, but after that they may need feeding every two hours or so, day and night, and even while sleepy they need changing every few hours.

If you have stitches or are very bruised, you can find yourself wishing that you were still pregnant, a thought that would have been incomprehensible only a day or two before. You can feel catapulted into motherhood before you are ready. You feel that you need time to recover yourself before taking on the 24-hour a day responsibility for a vulnerable baby, but unless you are very fortunate in your help this rarely happens. Even in hospital where you do have some expert assistance, the awareness of your baby's dependence on you can prevent you from relaxing and recuperating.

Unless you are prepared for it, you can be appalled to find that the reality after all the months of waiting can be an anti-climax, and that you may be one of the many mothers who go through a period of mourning for their vanished pregnancy and the baby that they imagined theirs was.

BOWELS

Constipation can figure even more prominently when you are newly delivered than in pregnancy, mainly because, if you have had an episiotomy, there is the anxiety about what will happen to your stitches when you do manage to open your bowels. Hospital with its routines, non-too private lavatories and often low standard of hygiene is not the ideal place to resolve the issue either. Many women find it is much better once they get home.

If you have had stitches, do not expect to go to the loo before at least the third day. When you think you can brave it, put a clean pad over your stitches to hold them in place. The stitches always do stand the strain, but it is hard to credit it at the time. Other ways of helping are to squat actually on the loo seat, to lubricate the rectum with a little baby cream and to practise your relaxation and breathing techniques at the time. It may help to lean to one side so that the pressure is off the stitch line. If the prospect is really terrifying, take painkillers beforehand.

Eating food with considerably more fibre than the average hospital diet will help too, but the problem most often is not that you feel no urge but that you dare not obey it. You could try the alternative remedies given for constipation in pregnancy (see p. 50) to see if they help the problem. Be careful not to take any purgatives such as senna, though, as they can be passed through the breast-milk and give the baby diarrhoea. A bulking laxative available on prescription and over the counter which will not affect the baby is Fybogel. Your midwife can supply suppositories or an enema if things get really bad.

Osteopathy can help if the problem becomes long-term which can happen, particularly after a forceps delivery.

PAINFUL COCCYX

The coccyx (tailbone) is displaced backwards when the baby passes through the birth canal. If it feels painful afterwards or even before the birth, take Hypericum.

REDUCING THE RISK OF INFECTION

Infection is a real risk in hospital — not surprising if you consider that you have a raw wound in your uterus where the placenta used to be. The opportunity for cross-infection is considerable where there is no disinfection of lavatories, bidets and baths between uses.

To avoid infection either have your baby at home or leave the hospital as soon as possible after the birth. If this is not possible, be scrupulous about changing your sanitary pad frequently and wiping yourself from front to back after emptying your bowels. Try to keep your stitches dry but do not share a hair-dryer and keep any contact with the loo seat to the minimum. Clean the bidet with disinfectant before using it or alternatively forgo using it altogether and either wash by pouring water over yourself while on the loo or bath two or three times a day. Use disinfectant on the loo seat, the water jug and the bath before using them.

EXCESSIVE BLEEDING

Bleeding can be quite profuse in the early days and gradually tails off as the days go by. The lochia, as it is called, is bright red initially and may contain clots, before slowly turning browny pink and eventually yellow. It can take as long as six weeks to stop altogether. When you become more active you may notice that the flow increases and becomes redder. If you get a real gush at any time, contact your midwife (see post-partum haemorrhage p. 112). You can control excessive lochia by applying pressure to a point just in from the webbing between the big toe and the one next to it on the upper side of the right foot or consult an acupuncturist.

RETAINED TISSUE

This can be allied to excessive bleeding. After birth your placenta and membranes will be examined closely to make sure that no part of them has been left behind. Small pieces of tissue may emerge with the lochia ordinarily, but tissue that is retained for any length of time can cause a problem. It may be responsible for continued bright red bleeding and can give rise to infection, signalled by an evil-smelling discharge and a rise in temperature. Treatment conventionally is by dilation and curettage, a gentle scraping-out of the contents of the uterus under general anaesthetic. An equally effective, but less invasive method is by treatment from an acupuncturist.

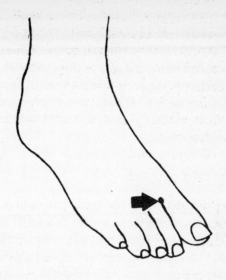

Acupressure point to stop excessive bleeding (Lochia)

Apply pressure to a point just in from the webbing between the big toe and its neighbour on the upper side of the right foot.

Seek help straight away if you start to feel fluey, have a rise in temperature or if your lochia starts to smell offensive. A course of antibiotics will probably be needed.

RETAINED PLACENTA

Left to itself the placenta should become detached from the wall of the uterus within half an hour of the birth. Sometimes you may need to give a push or two to help it on its way. However, it is standard practice to give an injection of Syntometrine into the thigh as the baby's shoulder is born. This is a combination of synthetic oxytocin and ergometrine, which stimulates the uterus to contract down hard within 7 minutes of administration. This reduces the likelihood of post-partum haemorrhage, but increases the possibility of the placenta becoming trapped inside the uterus. If this does happen, the placenta is usually removed manually under general, or occasionally epidural, anaesthetic. However the effect of the Syntrometrine wears off after two hours, so that waiting is an alternative to operative removal.

Patience may also be needed if you decline Syntometrine, as placentas sometimes take a while to become detached. If there is no excessive bleeding, there should be no need to do anything else. The cord can be cut once it has stopped pulsating. However waiting can get tedious and there are ways to speed things up.

Sometimes tension holds the placenta in and relaxing can let it go. A shot of pethidine or a cigarette may help, as can having a warm bath with your baby. Breast-feeding can stimulate the uterus to contract and expel the placenta and it helps to remain upright if at all possible. Drink raspberry leaf tea, squat and apply pressure to the acupressure point between and below the ankle bone and Achilles tendon on the inside of the right foot. Blowing hard into a bottle sometimes helps.

Homeopathic remedies

Try Caulophyllum and if it does not work, try Pulsatilla, but be patient — it might still take an hour for the placenta to appear.

Herbal remedies

Try ground ivy tincture, ½ to 1 teaspoonful (2.5–5 ml) under the tongue. Otherwise try 30–50 drops of angelica root — this can be combined with the labour tincture. An alternative remedy is 1 tablespoon of chopped balm leaves eaten raw. Or a large handful of feverfew leaves simmered in two cups of water for 3 minutes and steeped for 3 hours.

Acupuncture

Treatment by acupuncture can often be effective as shown in the following case of a home birth:

> We didn't want any complications so after what seemed like a long time of sitting on the bedpan, blowing into a bottle and putting the baby to the breast and the placenta still wouldn't deliver, I had acupuncture on the side of my foot and within minutes it came away.

Cranial osteopathy

A cranial osteopath was called to attend a woman who had given birth but whose placenta had not materialised. He worked on her head and said that it felt as though her sacrum had been pushed up under her ribs. As he held her head, he felt the sacrum suddenly fall back into position and the placenta came away immediately afterwards.

AFTERPAINS

These are the contractions of the shrinking uterus in the first week or two after the birth. They are not usually painful following the birth of a first baby, but do grow increasingly painful after each subsequent birth. They often coincide with breast-feeding and can be easily as intense as the contractions of labour.

Homeopathic remedy
Try Mag Phos.

Herbal remedies
Try taking 5–20 drops of motherwort tincture before feeding, or 10–30 drops catmint tincture, or 2 tablets of cramp bark, three times a day.

POST-NATAL DEPRESSION

Some depression is normal after having a baby. However well you may have prepared, you are bound to find that the reality of having a baby in your life quite a shock. It demands a huge adjustment in terms of your personal freedom and in the way that you and others see yourself.

However there is a point where the normal feelings of inadequacy, tiredness, anxiety and fearfulness about the baby can tip over into post-natal depression. This is an illness which is exclusive to women who have given birth. It may start immediately after the birth or take hold in the following weeks. It varies in severity, being easily recognised at its worst and perhaps missed in its lesser forms. It affects at least one in ten new mothers.

You may be able to diagnose the condition in yourself if you feel that you do not love your baby, that there is no point in getting up, that you are interested in nothing, and experience no emotions or feel unreal, strange or sad. You may find you have lost your sense of perspective, and are very tearful or hysterical, and feel overwhelmingly tired or panicky. You could dread going out, feel terrified, suicidal or worry that you are going mad. You may be waking early, unable to sleep or eat and take to obsessional or compulsive behaviour or feel very bored or angry. You may be depressed if you cannot manage to take the baby out of the house or cope with its most basic needs.

If you or your family think that post-natal depression is affecting you, it is important that you get help. One of the characteristics of the disease is, however, a refusal to admit to your problems, either because the state seems normal and warranted by the circumstances or because you fear the consequences and stigma of admitting to mental illness, and would prefer to recover by yourself. Time does cure it eventually, but in the meantime you are likely to be unable to enjoy all the pleasurable side of having a baby. You can get help through your health visitor or doctor. This may take the form of anti-depressants, a treatment which can be effective but which may have a time lag of two weeks before taking effect. Some doctors consider that the cause is hormonal and prescribe the synthetic hormone dydrogesterone which may correct the imbalance.

You can get effective treatment without ever consulting your doctor by trying one of the alternative therapies. This can prove satisfactory even when orthodox treatment has failed.

Self-help remedies
Post-natal depression may be prevented by eating the placenta. One woman who had suffered badly previously ate hers and found that she not only felt much better, and had no recurrence of her symptoms, but she actually looked a lot better, with supple skin and silky hair whereas previously her skin had become very dry and her hair had fallen out.

She did have a problem overcoming her natural revulsion and initially cooked pieces. She subsequently regretted this when she found that swallowing it raw was no more unpalatable, and likely to be more effective as steroids can be destroyed by heat. She kept the placenta in the fridge and cut off small squares and put them at the back of her mouth and swallowed them. She found it worked instantly as a natural antidepressant. You could try taking vitamin B6 and Efamol. Zinc is said to have very impressive results in improving post-natal depression.

Self-Heal Herbs sell a combination of herbs in capsule form for the treatment of depression or you could make your own brew according to Susun Weed's recipe in *The*

Wise Woman Herbal for the Childbearing Year. This uses:

½ oz (15 g) dried, shredded liquorice root
1 oz (25 g) dried, crumbled raspberry leaf
1 oz (25 g) dried, finely cut rosemary leaves
1 oz (25 g) dried, cut skullcap

Use 2 teaspoons of this mixture per cup of boiling water. Take two or more cups daily for as long as is needed.

Other sources of help include the Association for Post-Natal Illness, MAMA or the National Childbirth Trust, all of whom can provide you with a contact who has had PND and who has recovered from it (see Useful Addresses). This can give you the strength and support that you need to believe that you will recover too.

Post-natal depression is such a horrible condition that it might be better to consult a practitioner as soon as you can face it. Your partner may need to over-rule your objections if, as is likely, you are in no position to help yourself.

Cranial osteopathy
Cranial osteopaths believe that the illness is caused by the downward displacement of the uterus following birth and a resultant tug on the pituitary gland via the dura. Cranial osteopathy should be effective in helping the problem within two weeks.

Acupuncture
Chinese medicine believes that ten days rest in bed following the birth is essential for the prevention of post-natal depression. If you are depressed, though, you can be treated very successfully by acupuncture.

Homeopathic remedies
Post-natal depression rarely occurs after homeopathic births, but the remedies are as follows:

Simple blues, due to tiredness and excitement — Kali Phos.

More severe, with indifference, irritability and lack of maternal feelings, even rejection — Sepia.

Very despondent, changeable, weepy, worse in stuffy rooms, wants fresh air, better with sympathy — Pulsatilla.

Sad, irritable, cries on her own, worse with consolation — Natrum Muriaticum.

Listless, sad, exhausted, due to loss of fluids (ie haemorrhage or shock) — Phosphoric Acid.

Depression and exhaustion due to anaemia after haemorrhage — China.

Bach flower remedy
Try a combination of walnut, star of Bethlehem, mimulus (for fear), and rock rose (for panic).

11.
BREAST-FEEDING

There are two important things to remember about breast-feeding — the first is that correct positioning is vital, and the second is that you can do it if you really want to.

PREPARATION

Your breasts need little preparation for breast-feeding unless, unusually, one or both of your nipples turn inwards. In this case your midwife can supply you with breast shells which are worn in pregnancy and help to turn the nipple outwards. It can be a good idea to rub your nipples with a towel after a bath to make them slightly less sensitive because they can get sore when they suddenly come in for a lot of unaccustomed attention after delivery. You may notice quite early in the pregnancy that your nipples exude a yellow fluid. This is colostrum, the substance rich in protein and antibodies which the baby feeds off until the milk comes in. You do not need to express it but experimenting with your nipple and the areola, the brown area round the nipple, can give you an idea of where the baby's gums will need to go to get milk out.

Buy several good maternity bras. They are available from the National Childbirth Trust and department stores. It can be a relief to start wearing them as early as 5 months of pregnancy, because they are designed to give your breasts extra support.

STARTING TO FEED

It is easiest to put the baby to the breast as soon as it is

born, but it is possible that neither of you may feel like it
then. Your position is not so important for this first feed,
but it is important that the baby latches on correctly so
that it gets a proper feed and reduces the chances of you
developing nipple problems. Bring the baby to the breast
by putting your other hand behind its head. Persuade it to
open its mouth by stroking its chin with your nipple, and
then when it is open put the whole of the areola, *especially*
the lower side, into its mouth. The idea is that the baby
feeds from the breast, not the nipple, which should be well
back into the baby's mouth. The baby's suck exerts a
powerful vacuum and if this is mis-placed it can damage
the nipple, making feeding excruciatingly painful. If the
baby is on properly you will be able to see the muscles
beside its ear waggle as it feeds. The baby should be
allowed to feed for as long as it wants from the breast so
that it makes the decision about when to stop, but you can
detach it when necessary by inserting a finger into its
mouth. The milk flow can be stopped by depressing the
nipple.

Milk production is initiated by a change in hormones —
as the high level of oestrogen and progesterone fall
following the birth, the level of prolactin rises. Prolactin is
responsible for the formation of the milk so that at some
time between the second and fifth day your milk comes in.
This can happen quite suddenly within a few hours and
you may find that it means that your breasts alter
overnight from being soft and comfortable to becoming
rock-hard, hot and tender. They may also be enormously
swollen. This engorgement only lasts for a day or two
although it can be very uncomfortable for a while, and it
can cause problems if the baby finds it difficult to latch
on. It is at this time that the baby wakes up to the fact
that it feels hunger and it may start crying for food as
often as every two hours. This can be quite a taxing stage
in your new relationship so that it is important that you
rest and do not try to do anything other than get to know
each other.

A baby can be beautifully positioned but fail to get

enough milk if its mother does not 'let-down' her milk. The let-down reflex occurs when oxytocin is released from your brain. As a result the breasts start to tingle and tense and the nipple stands out, and shortly afterwards milk is ejected whether the baby is there or not. If this does not happen the baby will only get a little of the thirst-quenching thin blueish foremilk and none of the richer thicker hindmilk which contains more fat and which satisfies the baby's hunger. The reflex can be inhibited if you are feeling self-conscious or nervous or if you are dreading a further assault on your nipples. It can help to visualise milk spurting out or to concentrate on something lovable about the baby. If other people are putting you off, go elsewhere or ask them to leave. If you are afraid of feeding, you could try practising your relaxation and breathing techniques or try painkillers or alcohol.

The length of time for which a baby feeds for is not as important as letting the baby take what it wants. It should feed for as long as it wants on one side and may not need the other breast at that feed. Babies vary enormously in their enthusiasm and efficiency in feeding, but they all get quicker with practice. The important thing to remember is that breastfeeding is a question of supply and demand. The more often the baby demands milk by sucking on the breast, the greater the supply produced.

Your position

Frequent feeding can put a considerable strain on your back if it is not well supported because the ligaments are still soft from the pregnancy and can be easily damaged. Ideally you should sit in a chair with a high straight back and arms. You may need a cushion behind your back, and while the baby is very small, you should lie it on a pillow on your lap so that you do not have to bend over to feed it. Your back will ache badly if the baby is dragging on your breast as you feed or if you keep your head continually bent over and turned towards him or her. At night you may be able to feed while lying down in bed. The baby can be in any position so long as it is well-fixed and your back is supported.

SORE NIPPLES

Even if the baby is well-positioned, your nipples can become sore in the early days, which is hardly surprising when such a sensitive part of your body is suddenly subjected to intense wear. Do appreciate that it does get better and that it is worth persevering. Your nipples can be acutely painful and even cracked, but they have the power to heal quite rapidly, as they get increasingly less sensitive. There are ways of helping yourself through this stage, as follows:

- Use a nipple shield made of latex or silicone. There are two types of nipple protector. One looks like a Mexican hat and acts as an extra skin. The other has a rigid plastic casing with a teat on it, so that your milk is drawn out through the teat by suction alone and there is no pressure on your nipple from the baby's mouth. You can buy them from an NCT breast-feeding counsellor or a chemist. They have their disadvantages; it may take longer to feed, they need sterilising between feeds and if they are used for long the baby may reject the real thing. However if used sparingly, while feeding from the nipple as often as possible, they can be invaluable.
- Offer a dummy. Some babies just enjoy sucking and would be quite content to stay at the breast all day. If your baby is on for longer than you can stand, try giving it a dummy. They will make it quite clear when they want food rather than comfort-sucking, and you can discard it at around three months without difficulty.
- Avoid letting your nipples get soggy with leaked milk. Try allowing a drop of milk to dry on the nipple, being topless and exposing the nipples to air and sunlight or drying them with a hairdryer. Put a one-way nappy

liner next to your skin or make cages out of handle-less metal tea strainers inserted into your bra. You could try sitting a foot away from a 40 watt bulb with your nipples exposed to the heat several times a day.

- Try expressing milk by means of a pump (buy a syringe type or hire an electric one) and giving it to the baby in a bottle. This is a lot more work, but can provide a break which gives the nipple time to heal.
- Put something on to the nipple to help it heal, such as Hypercal, Calendula, Kamillosan or vitamin E ointment. You could also try crushed cucumber or if you are feeling strong, apply neat, fresh lemon juice. This stings dreadfully at first, but really seems to work. A more soothing effect can be had by mixing slippery elm bark powder together with warm water and putting the paste between squares of muslin inside your bra.
- Anaesthetise the nipple for the first few painful sucks by putting an ice cube on to it before starting to feed. If the pain gets worse during the feed, the baby may not be well-fixed, and it could be worth breaking off and starting again.

Homeopathic remedies

For simple soreness take Calendula internally and also use the mother tincture externally. If the nipples are sore, cracked and blistered, feel worse with warmth and at night, take Graphites. If the pain spreads from the nipple all over the body during feeding, if there are cracks especially on the right side, and feels worse with cold and damp, take Phytolacca.

NOT ENOUGH MILK

Even though you cannot completely empty a breast, there may be times when you feel that your baby is not getting enough. It is impossible to know exactly how much a breast-fed baby is taking, but if the baby's nappies are wet, its stools soft and yellow and it is gaining weight, then it is unlikely that the baby is not getting enough to eat overall. However there are times when they grow particularly fast and need more food, so that for a while you may feel that you do not have enough. The best remedy for insufficient milk is to keep on feeding. If you do that and do not short-circuit the demand-supply mechanism by giving complementary food, the supply should increase to match the baby's needs within a day or so.

If you are very active and do not eat adequately, you will find that your milk supply can start to fail. It is not indulgent to look after yourself when feeding, it is actually essential that you take some opportunity to rest, drink plenty of water, and eat three good meals plus snacks per day. If this seems a hopeless ideal reflect that the baby depends on your well-being for its growth and physical and mental development. This may make it easier to ask for help so that you can have at least one day's real rest. Guiness is also traditionally recommended for increasing the milk supply.

Herbal remedies
You can try drinking teas made from fennel, dill, anise, caraway or cumin. Vervain, borage and fenugreek are also noted for increasing your supply, while marshmallow, milkwort and lettuce improve the quality. Some herbalists recommend chewing liquorice root. Another suggestion is to take 4 tablespoons of 'brewers' yeast at lunch and supper-time or to try 10 drops of alfalfa tincture in water, four times a day until the milk increases.

Acupuncture
Consult an acupuncturist or try massaging the point just below the nail on the side of your little finger with another nail or matchstick.

Homeopathic remedies
In the absence of any other symptoms, Urtica Urens is

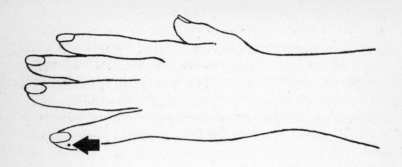

Acupressure point to increase the milk supply

Stimulate the point just below the nail on the side of your little finger with another nail or a matchstick.

worth trying as it will rebalance the supply in whichever direction necessary; it is particularly useful if there is no milk at all. Use nettle tea until you get the remedy. For a weak flow right from the beginning, associated with anxiety, fatigue and loss of sleep — Causticum. If the milk slows down or stops, you are weak, pale and maybe anaemic, take Agnus Castus. If the flow is very variable and changeable and you may feel the same, try Pulsatilla. Additional causes may be: acute emotional experience, take Natrum Muriaticum; sudden cold or damp, take Dulcemara or Pulsatilla; sensitivity — if feeding causes unbearable sexual excitement — try Calc Phos.

Self-help remedy
Finally there is a remedy which seems to work if you are really desperate to increase the milk supply. Known as sugar shock, it involves taking a large amount of sugar, at least 2 heaped tablespoonsful within one hour at the same time each day. It can be dissolved in lemon juice. It should work by stimulating the pituitary gland, and should be effective within a few days. If it has not worked within five days, abandon it.

Engorgement

Although your breasts will not stay engorged for more
than a day or two at the start of breast-feeding, they can
become engorged at any time thereafter if you have an
unusually long interval between feeds, for instance if the
baby sleeps longer than usual, or you are away from the
baby or when the baby is ill. Whatever the cause,
engorged breasts can be very uncomfortable indeed and
you may need to find some way of softening your breasts
so that baby can get the areola into its mouth.

It is important to have a bra that will expand when your
breasts are engorged because the swelling can add inches
to your dimensions. The National Childbirth Trust does
one with laces and another with an extra hooked piece at
the back.

The first remedy is to feed as often as possible and keep
the breasts comfortable this way. You may need to
express some milk first in order to soften the breast so
that the baby can latch on, which is impossible if the
breast is completely hard. This can be done by getting on
to all fours in the bath or by hanging over a basin so that
your breasts dangle over it, and splashing or spraying
them with warm water. This should help the milk to shoot
out in thread-like jets.

You might prefer to save the milk for later on, as within
a couple of weeks the supply will be adjusted to the baby's
needs and it will be less abundant. You can express by
means of a syringe-type or electrical pump and store it in
the freezer in small sterilised bottles. You can also save it
by catching the drips from the breast not in use in
specially designed shells. It is important to freeze it
straight after the feed so that the milk does not
accumulate bacteria.

Other ways of helping lessen the swelling include
putting chilled cabbage leaves inside your bra, and
stroking the swelling from the nipple outwards. You need
to handle your breasts carefully as they can easily be
bruised when they are engorged.

TOO MUCH MILK

Although the problem of having too much milk does not cause anxiety, it can be very inconvenient if you go on leaking milk, flooding the bed and soaking your clothes well past the early weeks. You can freeze the excess milk (see under 'Engorgement') or donate it to a human milk bank. The feeding sister at your local maternity unit will be very grateful for any contributions of milk, however small, with which to feed very tiny and sick babies.

If you really want to reduce the amount of milk you produce, try drinking teas of sage of herb robert. Also if you have too much milk, your breasts are hard and hot, and you are not thirsty — take one dose of Belladonna 6 hourly until there is an improvement.

BLOCKED DUCT OR MASTITIS

Sometimes one of the milk ducts in the breast may become blocked. It can happen if you wear clothes that constrict your breasts or if your arm presses on to the breast. It results in pain in one specific area which may become reddened and be tender and hard to the touch. If you do nothing about it, your temperature may rise and you will feel ill.

Start taking action at the first hint of tenderness or hardness. Encourage the baby to feed frequently on that side and use a pump gently if it does not feel empty after feeding. While feeding or using the pump, stroke the hardened part towards the nipple — your partner can help with this — and vary the baby's position so that it is exerting the most suction on the blockage. Try having a hot bath and using a fine-toothed comb on your soapy breast to urge the lump out to your nipple. Swinging your arm round and round can improve the blood supply to the breast. Heather Welford in her book *A-Z of Feeding in the First Year* suggests placing a hot water bottle wrapped in a towel next to the tender area, if feeding is painful.

You can take 1 g of vitamin C and 6–8 garlic perles

every three hours to combat infection or try two echinacea tablets every two hours. If you use the tincture use $\frac{1}{2}$ a drop per pound of body weight per dose. Repeat the dose up to six times a day if you have a fever and continue taking it two to three times a day for seven days after the problem has eased.

If there is no improvement or you get worse, you may need antibiotics. There is no need to stop feeding, but remind your doctor that you are breast-feeding if he or she prescribes them. Take lactobacillus with them if you ever suffer from thrush.

Aromatherapy
Try a compress of a drop of rose, geranium and lavender oils in cold water.

Homeopathic remedies
If there is a sudden problem, take Aconite within the first 24 hours. If the breast is hard and perhaps hot, but the skin is not red, the breast is sensitive to touch and movement, and maybe worse on the left, take Bryonia. If the breast is hard, hot, red, painful and extremely sensitive to touch and movement, and you feel restless, take Belladonna. If the pain is on the right and you are pale, not hot but are perspiring, try Calcarea Carbonica. When the breast is very hard and sensitive and is worse on the right, take Phytolacca. If an infection or abscess is indicated, as with a raised temperature and the problem is worse with warmth, worse at night and you are perspiring, try Mercurius. When there are hard lumps in the breast and you feel worse in the cold or damp, and the nipple may be retracted, use Silica. With stinging and burning, a cracked nipple, which is worse with the warmth of the bed and washing, and you crave fresh air, take Sulphur. If there are splinter-like pains, hypersensitivity and sweating and are much worse in the cold, take Hepar Sulph.

PART THREE

CARING FOR YOUR BABY

12.
YOU AND YOUR BABY

At some time after the birth — either hours of days — you will find yourself in charge of your new baby. This can be a moment of great triumph, but it may also be tempered with anxiety. Even if you are used to handling small babies, assuming full responsibility for your own can be daunting.

New parents are typically and understandably anxious about their new babies. They lack the experience with that particular child which is necessary for them to be able to feel confident about the way it is behaving. They are often unable to anticipate its needs, work out why it is crying or have any idea of how it will behave in the next 24 hours. Babies are unpredictable and demanding, and although most babies will have settled down by the time they are three months old, the difficulties can seem overwhelming in those first few weeks of life.

Babies are in fact very tough and can survive quite considerable neglect, as demonstrated by the babies who lived for six days after the Mexican earthquake without any attention at all. In fact a certain amount of neglect, such as that a second or subsequent child suffers by virtue of its place in the family, is healthy. However it takes time for you to be that relaxed about your baby and there are no short-cuts to gaining experience.

Make the most of the chance to absorb yourself in your first child, as it will not come again. Remember, though, that you are not the only person in the world who can look after it, so accept offers of help and take the opportunity to go out or do something for yourself. It can be easy to feel that everything you do is connected with the baby —

and they do take up an enormous part of every day — and this can cause an undercurrent of resentment. It is quite normal to feel that you as an individual are being lost, that your interests are over-looked and that you are now only X's mother. Again this should only be a brief stage, but handing the baby over from time to time can make it seem much briefer.

CARE OF THE UMBILICUS

The cord will have been cut and clamped with string, elastic or a plastic clamp. The clamp is released after a few hours, and then it is a matter of a few days before the stump of the cord dries up and drops off. Because there is a risk of the umbilicus becoming infected (greater in hospital), the stump is usually swabbed with surgical spirit and dusted with antistaphylococcal powder. Some midwives have discovered that it heals best and the cord comes off most quickly if it is cleaned with water alone, and the baby is bathed frequently.

Alternatively you can dress the stump with honey which is a natural antiseptic or dry it up with witch hazel. Calendula powder is useful for healing. It is important to stop the nappy knocking the stump while it is healing. Your midwife will not discharge the baby from her care until the stump is off.

JAUNDICE IN NEW BABIES

Some jaundice is very common in new babies and shows itself by turning the baby's skin and the white of its eyes yellow, often giving the baby the appearance of a healthy tan. Usually jaundice starts between the second and third day, and it is caused when the liver breaks down the extra red blood cells that are no longer needed once the baby is breathing and taking in its own oxygen. The cells are broken down and converted into, among other products, bilirubin, which is fat-soluble and needs to be made water-soluble so that it can be excreted. If this does not occur, the bilirubin remains and gathers in fatty tissue — under the skin staining it yellow, and around the kidneys. Occasionally it collects around the basal ganglia of the brain and this can lead to kernicterus if the jaundice is not treated, a condition which causes brain damage. If the baby's colour deepens and it seems lethargic, blood will be taken to ensure that its bilirubin levels are not rising too high.

Orthodox treatment consists of putting the baby under special lights. You can try a home version by exposing the baby to sunlight and natural light by putting its crib under the window.

Jaundice is more common in babies whose mothers have been given Syntometrine of Syntocinon.

Alternative remedies include drinking at least two cups of catmint or dandelion tea daily, and giving Nat Phos tissue salt 6x to the baby.

Another suggestion is that of giving the baby molasses water (one teaspoon molasses to one cup of cooled boiled water) by dropper after each food until the milk comes in.

SLEEP

In the early weeks the baby cannot be expected to sleep to any particular pattern or to recognise night from day, although some do. Sometimes you will find that they have periods of activity at the same time as they did before they were born.

One way to encourage sleep at night is to make it clear to the baby that it is not a playtime. Feed the baby when necessary and change it if essential, but don't talk to it or play with it. Keep the light down and put the baby back into its crib as soon as possible. If it is cold, put a hot water bottle out of your bed into the crib when you take the baby out, so that it is warm when you put the baby back. Playing a long-playing musical box after the feed so that the baby comes to associate the sound with going to sleep is sometimes effective. Alternatively a tape of uterine sounds may help both of you to get back to sleep after being woken. Having the baby's crib beside your bed means that you can feed it without fully waking.

A few babies sleep through the night by the time they are six weeks old, but most do not and may not for many months yet. Firm handling and a routine can help, and there is a case for saying that if you do not respond to night crying for food, the baby will stop demanding it within a week. This is only recommended for babies of 12 lb (6 kg) or more, and is hard to do, although it does seem to work.

As with everything else, babies vary in their need for sleep, some being almost permanently asleep and others hardly ever shutting their eyes. A non-sleeper is very much harder work because you get much less chance to sleep or do anything for yourself. A baby like this may develop into the type of adult that needs little sleep, but the problem can also be caused by allergy (see p. 154) or the torsion on the brain caused by the pressures exerted at birth. In this case, cranial osteopathy can work brilliantly so that a child may start sleeping normally within a day of the treatment.

Avena Sativa Comp. which is a combination of oats, hops, passion flower and valerian, can be taken by mothers and children. It is said to be a natural aid to peaceful relaxation and particularly useful after a stressful day. To aid sleep take 10-20 drops in a little water half an hour before retiring. Repeat the dose if necessary. Children should be given half the adult dose.

Acupressure may also work well; an acupunturist will show you the technique of rubbing the acupuncture points relevant to your baby.

Baby massage given an hour or two before expected periods of restlessness or sleeplessness may help to soothe the baby and improve the problem. You can find out how best to do it by taking the baby to someone who specialises in baby massage (contact the Active Birth Movement for details of practitioners) or consulting the books mentioned in the booklist. You could start with the massage movement known as Harmonising Fire and Water described on p. 163.

It is best to avoid sedating the baby if possible, although it is tempting to hope that it may break the cycle of non-sleeping and give you a well-earned rest. This is because the drugs often work in reverse making the baby even more active and less likely to sleep. With a toddler patterns of sleeplessness can often be broken by sending the child to spend the night with relations or a friend.

WEANING

You need not start weaning your breast-fed baby until it is at least six months old, providing that you are eating well and the baby is gaining weight. Growth spurts occur at around three weeks, six weeks and three months, and the increased demand at these times may make you feel that you are not providing enough milk and query the need for solid food. If you keep breast-feeding, the milk supply will have increased to cope within 48 hours, although in the meantime the baby may seem hungry and wake more often.

When you start introducing solid foods, it is best to introduce one food at a time and delay the introduction of milk, wheat, and eggs. If you have a family history of allergy or if the baby has shown any hint of an allergic response, such as colic, eczema or asthma, you might want to start your baby on the following weaning diet suggested by Dr Cant and Janet Bailes of St George's Hospital, London.

Start by introducing food in the order given below, offering it daily for a week, and watching carefully to see if it causes a skin rash or loose watery stools. If there is a reaction avoid the food for several months.

1. Milk-free baby rice (check the label on the packet) mixed with water or expressed milk.
2. Puréed root vegetables, such as potatoes, carrots, parsnips, swede, turnips.

3. Puréed fruit, such as apple, pear, banana, but no citrus fruits until the baby is 9 months old.
4. Other vegetables, such as peas, beans, lentils, broccoli, etc.
5. Other cereals — but no wheat until the baby is 8 months old.
6. Lamb, turkey and then the other meats.
7. Fish — but not until 10 months.
8. Other milk and milk products — but not before 10 months. If the baby is having less than four feeds a day, you may need to give soya milk. Start with yoghurt, boiled cow's milk and then if these are tolerated, introduce cheese, butter, etc.
9. Eggs — but not until 1 year.

13.
ILLNESS IN BABIES — WHAT TO DO

As you get to know your child, you will develop the intuition that tells you when it is not well, and whether the illness is serious or not. At first however you will not know your baby's individual behaviour patterns well enough to do this, and babies behave unpredictably even when perfectly well, so that in the early days you are likely to have lots of alarms about its health. This is not necessarily a bad thing; some degree of anxiety is useful and even experienced mothers feel the need for extra caution with their new babies.

Illness in babies is a bit like labour — you can be certain if it is the real thing but it is less easy to be sure if it only might be. When the child is older you will know what you can treat yourself and what requires medical attention, but in the meantime the following guidelines may be helpful.

SERIOUS ILLNESS — TAKE ACTION STRAIGHT AWAY

- Fits, convulsions, not breathing, unconsciousness.
- Difficulty in breathing, grunting, rapid breathing.
- Being blue or very pale.
- Unexplained bleeding from any part of the body.
- Stiff neck and irritability.

SIGNS OF ILLNESS

Watch out for these signs of illness and seek medical help when necessary.

- The child is unusually hot or cold, test by kissing its forehead. Bear in mind that young babies can be quite ill with a normal or lowered temperature. A raised temperature may mean that the hands and feet are cold when the forehead is hot. If the baby's temperature is up, take any clothes off and keep the child cool by sponging with tepid water or using a fan if the temperature rises above 102°F (39.4°C).
- The baby refuses more than one feed or meal.
- A blocked nose prevents the baby from feeding.
- Continual or unusual screaming or crying.
- The child is obviously in pain.
- Frequent vomiting or diarrhoea. This is particularly serious in little children because they can quickly become dehydrated.
- The child refused to smile. A child can sound very ill with a hacking cough, but be all right if it is able to smile, eat and play. A sick child gives all these things up and is either very fretful and unhappy, or spends a lot of time sleeping.

If you take your child to a doctor, there are certain questions you should ask about your child's illness:

1. What is the diagnosis? This can be useful to know for the future. However, often there is not any positive diagnosis, just that the child is ill but not seriously and will probably get better without treatment.
2. What is the treatment? Not all childhood illnesses require antibiotics, but if you are given medicines take notes of the dosage and if there are likely to be any side effects. Ask about alternatives too.
3. How soon will it be before the child is likely to improve?
4. Are there any signs you should look out for that might suggest the child was getting worse?
5. When should you bring the child back if there is no improvement?
6. How long is the child likely to be infectious (if applicable)?

Trust your instinct and be persistent if you think there is
something really wrong.

WHEN TO CALL THE DOCTOR

Make sure before the baby is born that you are registered
with a doctor with whom you are happy, because
consultation rates can rise dramatically once you have a
small baby. Word of mouth is the best way of finding one
— ask other mothers whom they recommend. Some
doctors are happy for you to talk to them before
registering. You can register the baby with a docter other
than your own if you wish, but there may be some
advantages to having the same doctor for the whole
family. Doctors who have young children themselves may
be the most sympathetic and understanding. You need to:

- Check that you can consult your doctor by phone,
  bearing in mind that this puts pressure on them to
  visit you if your child sounds ill, even if you have not
  asked for a visit.
- Be sure that they do night calls themselves.
- Ensure that they will see a sick child the same day in
  surgery.

It is quicker to take your child to the surgery to be seen
than to ask a doctor to call. It is usually safe to take a
child with a fever to the surgery by car, although you
should let the receptionist know if you think your child is
infectious. Put your baby in clothes that undo easily and
take a spare nappy.

If you have difficulty in deciding whether to call the
doctor — and it is usually in the early hours of the
morning that this seems to be the greatest problem —
consider how you would advise a friend in the same
situation, or if you would drive the child to hospital or
drive miles to an open chemist if necessary. A good doctor
would rather you called unnecessarily than fail to call
when you think that something is wrong. If your child is
suddenly and seriously ill or has a bad accident, ring for

an ambulance or take him or her to the nearest accident and emergency unit. Make sure you know how to get there before you need it.

FIRST AID

Small babies tend to have fewer accidents than children, although there is a first time for each advance they make, as many a mother has discovered when her baby rolled off the changing mat. However they soon grow into an extremely accident-prone phase, where you have to anticipate their every move.

There are some alternative remedies that work incredibly well, which are well worth keeping in a first aid box for the inevitable accident. Arnica or A B C tablets administered after any serious fall or bang are very effective, and both you and the child may benefit from Rescue Remedy if the accident has given a shock. Take 4 drops of the remedy in water or drop directly into the mouth. Nelsons offer a range of creams or ointments which provide rapid and effective treatment for a number of minor ailments, including bruising — applied straight away the treatment removes the pain and stops the bruise developing, though avoid putting it on broken skin; and burns — hold the area that has been burned or scalded under cold running water for 10 minutes and then apply the ointment all over and around the area. This eases the pain and prevents blistering. Hypercal and calendula are good for healing cuts and sores and can be very good for skin complaints. There is also a pyrethrum spray for bites and stings which is very effective.

INFECTIOUS DISEASES

Babies may be less likely to pick up the common childhood diseases because they retain a certain immunity from their mothers for the first six months or so. This may mean that if they do come into prolonged contact with a disease because an older brother or sister has it, they may only get it very mildly. Some diseases such as whooping cough and measles can be very serious in babies, when they are too young to be immunised against them, so it is very important to make sure you avoid contact with known cases when you have a baby.

Rubella (German measles)
Incubation period 14-21 days. It starts as a flat pink rash beginning behind the ears and giving rise to enlarged glands at the back of the neck. Generally mild but keep away from pregnant women who have not been immunised. This is only likely to apply to first pregnancies as non-immune women are immunised after birth. Blood is tested for immune status when you start ante-natal care.

Measles
Incubation period 10-15 days. Starts as a bad cold with a cough and red eyes and perhaps a fever. Look for white spots on the inside of the cheeks. After a few days dark red spots cover the body and the child develops a high fever, may have no appetite and seem very ill. There can be complications of bronchitis, ear infections and — more rarely — inflammation of the brain. The child is no longer infectious once the symptoms have gone. A homeopathic prophylaxis, preventing the child contracting the disease, is to give Pulsatilla 30 daily from the third day after contact until the fifteenth or sixteenth day when the danger of infection will have passed. If measles develops contact a homeopath although you may find Bryonia helpful generally and Euphrasia should help inflamed eyes and eyelids. See p. 169 to treat the high fever that often accompanies measles.

Whooping cough
Incubation period 7-10 days. Starts as a cough and cold and then develops the typical whoop although this may not be present in babies. The cough takes the child by surprise so that they are forced to cough before taking a

breath. Each prolonged cough may end in vomiting. Whooping cough is said to be non-infectious 28 days from the start of symptoms, but the cough may last longer. A homeopathic prophylaxis is to give your baby three doses of Pertussin 30 at any time after it is six months old. Give one dose one night, one the following morning and then one that night. If the child is in contact with whooping cough give one dose of Pertussin 30 once a week for three weeks. It should only be given to babies under three months in consultation with a homeopath.

If the child does get whooping cough it would be as well to seek help from a homeopath. The following remedies should prove helpful. Give Drosera for whooping cough with spasms of coughing which follow on top of each other and result in gagging and vomiting, or if the cough is worse at night and when the child lies down. For a suffocating cough which makes the child stiff and blue in the face and results in vomiting of phlegm, give Ipecac. Consult a homeopathic pharmacy about the use of Pertuderon 1 and 11 which can be very helpful in alleviating symptoms.

Chicken pox
Incubation period about 14 days. Starts with spots that soon become clear blisters which get knocked off and become pustules which soon turn to scabs. Not a particularly serious illness, but can cause severe itching. It is no longer infectious once the spots have turned to scabs.

To prevent itching, add 4 drops of peppermint oil to a bath, and dap spots with diluted distilled witch hazel, or calamine lotion available from a chemist.

Mumps
Incubation period about 21 days. Starts with the gland in front of the ear swelling and becoming tender. One or both sides may be affected. The child may have difficulty in drinking and eating. The child is infectious for 7 days after the swelling has gone down.

Try minute doses of poke root tincture, ½ ml, three times a day.

Tetanus

Homeopathic prophylaxis (need not be given in the first year unless you live in the country) consists of two doses of Hypericum 200 per week for one month.

Diphtheria

This is very rare nowadays but you can protect your child from the disease by giving Diphtherium 30 once a week for four to six weeks.

IMMUNISATION

This is a controversial issue upon which you will have to make up your own mind after enquiring about all the facts both for and against. It is a decision that parents often agonise about. Some homeopaths believe that fighting the common childhood illnesses with immunisation supressing them makes the child weaker.

If you decide not to have your child immunised, you may want to ask a homeopath about prophylactic remedies in an epidemic. If your child does contract one of the diseases, it can be treated homeopathically to reduce its length and strength, for example whooping cough treated homeopathically only lasts seven days.

If you do choose to get the immunisations done, the ill-effects can be minimised by giving Arnica or Thuja 30 beforehand.

14.
AN A–Z OF COMMON INFANT COMPLAINTS AND THEIR REMEDIES

ALLERGIES

There seems to be an increase in the number of babies and children experiencing allergic reactions either to their food or something in their environment. You might suspect allergy if your baby is unusually fretful, has diarrhoea or constipation, is particularly thirsty, sleeps little or fitfully, has a body rash (see eczema p. 168) or frequent nappy rash (see p. 170), is colicky (see p. 159), seems to have a perpetual cold, has dark rings under its eyes or has puffy swelling around them.

Very susceptible babies (those with one or both parents with an allergy themselves) can react to minute traces of your food in your breast milk. They may react very badly to formula milk (see p. 145 weaning). Fruit juices and vitamin drops can also cause problems. It can help to identify the cause if you make a chart of the baby's food intake and subsequent responses.

Babies can also react to the things in contact with their skin. This might be wool, or the washing powder or fabric conditioner using in washing clothes and bedding (see nappy rash), or it could be the soap, baby bath liquid, shampoo, lotion or wipes used in cleaning the baby. Eliminate the cause and wash with water alone, or ask your doctor to prescribe Oilatum, a liquid emulsion which is put into bath water and cleans without damaging the skin.

Wheezy babies may be reacting to the house dust mite which lives in dust and bedding. If your child is unlucky enough to suffer like this, you may find the condition improves with scrupulous attention to daily vacuuming and damp dusting. The Asthma Society can give details (see p. 182).

Allergic children should be under the supervision of a doctor, although they are not all open-minded about the diagnosis. Food-allergic children should be seen by a dietician; your GP can refer you to a community dietician.

You may want to consider eating a low-allergen diet yourself if you are pregnant and think your baby is likely to be allergic to food. There is no real evidence yet that this will prevent the baby acquiring allergies, but it is thought to help. You will need dietary advice.

Eliminating the cause of the problem may be sufficient to ensure your child's health but also consider constitutional treatment from a homeopath for you or the baby. Acupressure can have a dramatic effect on allergic children, reducing the sensitivity overnight.

ASTHMA

This may start as a nocturnal cough and frequent colds. You should have it diagnosed by a medical practitioner, but you can have it treated by a homeopath or osteopath.

BURNS

See section on first aid, p. 150. If the burns are severe, give Cantharis to prevent infection.

CHEST INFECTIONS

Babies can have horrible-sounding coughs and yet not be seriously ill. Sometimes, though, the cough may not sound particularly bad, but the infection will have travelled down the respiratory tract so that it is described as being 'on the chest' and therefore potentially more serious. It can be hard to decide by yourself if this has occurred, although you can listen to your baby's chest without a stethoscope by putting your ear to its chest or back. It is a good idea to have babies with a cough checked medically, although older children are unlikely to be ill in this way without a fever or seeming sick in other ways.

Breast-fed babies can be treated for infection through their mothers. Echinacea is an effective anti-microbial herb, which works for both viruses and bacteria. Use 1-2 teaspoonsful of the root in a cupful of water, simmered for 15 minutes. Drink three times a day. Maintain the treatment for at least seven days, even when the condition is improved.

Sometimes a chest infection leads to breathing difficulties such as wheezing, being unable to suck enough air in or out, breathing much faster than 40 breaths a minute, which may result in the baby turning blue or the lower ribs or the skin at the neck being sucked in. Any of these signs are an indication for seeking help straightaway.

Frequent night coughs and attacks of wheezy bronchitis may be an indication of asthma (see p. 155) in susceptible children.

Homeopathic remedies
Give ABC (a combination of Aconite, Belladonna and Chamomilla) which is useful at the start of any childhood illness. For a dry painful cough, try Bryonia. For a barking cough or a constant tickling cough, try Drosera. For a cough with coarseness and loss of voice, try Phosphorus.

CHOKING

It is terrifying to find your child choking and turning blue from lack of breath. Make sure you know what to do in case it happens.

If the problem is caused by food obstructing the airway,

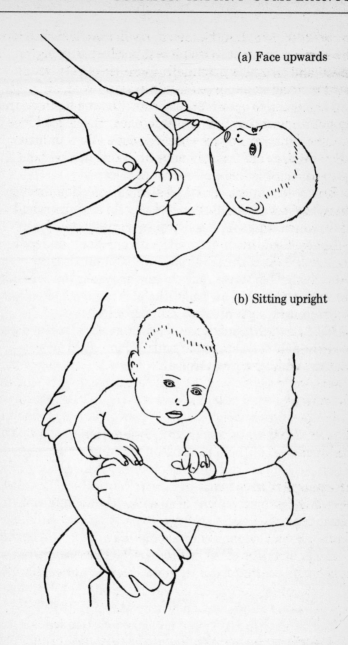

(a) Face upwards

(b) Sitting upright

The Heimlich manoeuvre

or by fluid having been inhaled, try holding the child upside-down and banging it three or four times on the back between the shoulder blades. If this doesn't work, try the following steps.

Lie the child down face upwards. Put one hand on the child's abdomen so that the heel of it is on the spot just above the navel and below the rib cage. Put your other hand over the first one. Then push the abdomen with a quick upward thrust and repeat as necessary.

This type of resuscitation, known as the Heimlich manoeuvre, can also be done with child sitting upright or on your knee. In this case wrap your arms around the child from behind, make a fist with one hand and place it thumbside in, at the point on the abdomen already described. Then press quickly upward as before. The upward pressure of air below the obstruction should force it out. If it fails get medical help urgently.

Take Rescue Remedy yourself for shock afterwards, and give it or Aconite to the child. If the child is bruised by the procedure, give Arnica.

COLDS

The more babies are exposed to other people, the greater the likelihood of them picking up a cold or cough, even when very small. Babies with older brothers or sisters will be exposed to them from the start. You will feel happier if people with obvious colds keep away from your new baby, but it is unrealistic to isolate your baby totally, so your baby is likely to get one sometime.

Colds in babies often last two weeks or more, and can seem to be continual during the winter. In most cases the child might be fretful, may wake more often and can have problems in feeding, but they are not seriously ill.

You can help a baby with a blocked nose to feed by removing the mucus with a dropper or by mouth. Decongestant drops from the chemist can help, but they must be used sparingly as they become ineffective within a few days. You can also make breathing easier by rubbing

Vick on the chest, or by putting a drop of eucalyptus oil or the liquid contents of a Karvol capsule on to the sheet at the head end.

Some children respond well to a Wrights' vapouriser, available from the chemists. This consists of a little tin containing a night light which heats a porous stone soaked in a pungent coal tar liquid. When it is lit, the fumes fill the air and reach the baby's lungs.

Central heating can make things worse by drying the atmosphere. You can increase the humidity by putting wet towels over the radiators or using a humidifier.

If your child always has a streaming nose, it would be worth thinking about whether the cause was not in fact a cold, but an allergy (see p. 154). Colds can cause real problems if they result in middle ear or chest infections (see p. 155).

Homeopathic remedies
Give Aconite two to three times on the first day of a cold. For a sneezy cold with a nose running like a tap, try Nat Mur. For fluey colds, try Gelsemium. For a feverish head cold, try Merc. Sol.

COLIC

Colic is a horrible problem which sometimes afflicts small babies. It can start at any time after birth and typically lasts for three months. It can strike at any time of the day or night and often occurs at the same time each evening. It causes the baby to start crying suddenly and with a desperate intensity, giving every appearance of being in acute pain. It often comes in spasms which make the baby arch its back or draw its knees up to its chest. The attacks can last an hour or more, and subside gradually leaving the baby and parents exhausted. It can be agonising to see your tiny baby in agony and be unable to help it. You start by feeling deeply sorry for the infant, but as the crying continues you can become maddened by it so that you would do anything to stop it.

Colic does usually pass with time and it does not appear to do the baby any lasting damage. Its causes are not fully understood, although it does seem to be connected with the immaturity of the baby's digestive system. It often ends as abruptly as it started at around 13 weeks. You can just sit it out or try some of the following remedies, although it is possible that only time will help. There are lots of remedies — which perhaps reflects the degree of despair to which colic can drive parents.

During an attack the baby may be calmed by being held over the shoulder and walked around. A dummy can be a god-send even if you have to hold it in, because the sucking instinct will sometimes win over the need to cry. Some babies feel better if they are held on your lap on their tummies, and heat from a warm hot water bottle (not hot) on the tummy helps too. A tape of uterine sounds which is played loudly by the baby's head can make a great difference, and some people think that giving a spoonful of boiled water before a feed helps. You may find that adding Rescue Remedy to the water makes a considerable difference.

The colic may be cured or lessened by a change in the baby's milk. Many colicky babies are allergic either to their formula milk or some constituent of their mother's breast-milk. A bottle-fed baby may be better on soya milk, and a breast-fed baby may improve if you give up eating possible allergens, especially milk and egg. This is because tiny particles of these proteins are present in your milk as little as two hours after eating them and sensitive babies may react to them with colic or eczema, diarrhoea and vomiting. Try eliminating the following common allergens from your diet for a week. If there is no improvement, do not continue with it, but if there is, start by introducing the foods singly leaving at least two days between each kind, so that you can monitor the baby's reaction. You MUST be scrupulous about excluding the forbidden foods.

- Milk in any form, ie butter, cheese, cream, yoghurt, skimmed milk powder (can also be found in processed

food as sodium caseinate, caseinate, whey or non-fat milk solids).
- Eggs (also yolk, white, lactalbumin and egg lecithin).
- Wheat, including bread and any of the many products that include wheat flour.
- Chocolate and cocoa, even milk-free.
- Citrus fruits and tomatoes.
- Beef and poultry.
- Any other food or drink that seems to give your baby colic. It may help to keep a food diary and a chart of the crying spells.

If the baby does respond to dietary measures, it might be wise to delay weaning as long as possible and to avoid the above foods when you do start (see p. 145).

Herbal remedies
The remedies can be passed through the breast-milk or given directly to the baby. You can drink decoctions of dill, fennel or the bruised seeds of aniseed, or eat coriander leaves or ginger, either fresh or cooked. You could give the baby a teaspoonful of dill, catmint or chamomile tea.

Cranial osteopathy
This can help some babies by freeing their cranial base and relieving distortions of the skull which may be causing pressure on the vagus nerve leading to gastric irritation.

Mohammed had cried almost from the moment of his forceps birth. He had bad attacks of colic lasting up to an hour after almost every feed and at six weeks his parents were getting desperate. He was taken to a cranial osteopath who treated him for about 40 minutes. He seemed to enjoy the treatment, settling down and going to sleep. He released a lot of wind from his bowel and seemed calmer when he woke up. He went back for further treatments and gradually the colic improved.

Massage

There are particular techniques of massage to help babies with colic and other problems. Regular massage is considered beneficial for all babies. You can find out about the techniques by reading the booklet *Massage for Life* by Stephen Russell and Yehudi Gordon.

Acupuncture

An acupuncturist can help improve your baby's colic. You may be able to help yourself by exerting pressure between the baby's first and second toe, at a point a finger's breadth from the base. This will calm the liver, relax the muscles and reduce inflammation.

Homeopathic remedies

It is preferable if a baby suffering from colic is seen by a trained homeopath so that an individual diagnosis and treatment can be made. The names of qualified homeopaths practising in your area can be obtained from either The British Homeopathic Association or The Society of Homeopaths (see Useful Addresses).

Aromatherapy

Try dipping a small towel in warm water to which a few drops of chamomile oil have been added, wringing it out and placing over the baby's stomach.

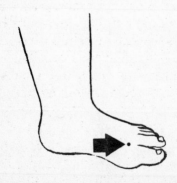

Acupressure point for easing colic

Finally, you yourself will need help and support through a troubled time. Your health visitor may be able to give practical support or you may find that speaking to someone from Cry-sis makes you feel better. This is a voluntary organisation run by mothers, all of whom have suffered with crying babies (see Useful Addresses).

CONSTIPATION

This is only a problem if passing infrequent stools causes the baby distress. Some breast-fed babies go for days without a dirty nappy and it causes them no discomfort. Bottle-fed babies are more likely to have bulky, hard stools which can be difficult to pass. If you think the baby needs some help because it is uncomfortable, you could give it some diluted prune juice or try taking syrup of figs or eat prunes or figs yourself.

Homeopathic remedies
If the rectum is inactive so that the baby has to strain to pass a soft stool and can only do so when there is a large accumulation, give Alumina. If the problem persists consult a homeopath.

Baby massage
Can relieve constipation and also works for colic, indigestion, vomiting and diarrhoea. Stephen Russell recommends a series of Taoist massage patterns in his book *Massage for Life*. This one, known as Harmonising Fire and Water is the first of eight patterns which are good for releasing tensions in the abdomen. This should be done preferably at a quiet time and with the baby naked. Using as much pressure as would smooth a crumpled piece of tissue paper without tearing it, stroke the baby. Start at the midline of the chest using the fingers of both hands, move down the torso to the pubic bone, then separate the hands to the sides of the torso and pull up into the armpits. Circle over the breast region and meet again on the midline at the chest. This balances the heart and the

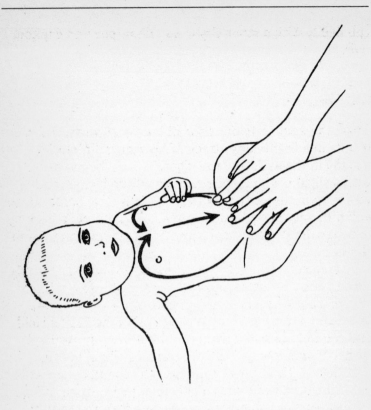

Baby massage for colic, constipation, indigestion, vomiting and diarrhoea

kidneys. Do this for up to twenty one cycles, each lasting ten seconds. It should be done with great sensitivity and delicacy to achieve the best results. It builds physical and emotional stability, helps to calm a hyperactive child, relaxes the chest and strengthens the digestive system.

CRADLE CAP

This is a kind of thick, scaly dandruff which often forms on the scalp and eyebrows of babies. To get rid of it, dab the affected area with olive oil (not baby oil which is mineral and which can be damaging to the skin), allow the scales to soften for a couple of hours or longer, and then rub firmly with a rough dry towel. Shampoo and dry the hair.

CROUP

This is an acute inflammation of the vocal cords, which results in a frightening attack of breathing difficulties, usually in the middle of the night. The child goes to bed with a slight cold, maybe sounding a little hoarse, and wakes up in the early hours with a distinctive harsh cough and difficulty in sucking in enough air. Your child is likely to be terrified — and so are you, but it is important not to show it.

Humidity helps so that the thing to do is to boil a kettle continuously in the bedroom, so that the air fills with steam. You can make a tent with sheets to concentrate the steam as long as you are careful with the kettle. Hold and comfort child and there should be an improvement within 15 minutes, so that you can all go back to bed.

If there is no improvement, or if the condition seems to be getting worse and the child cannot settle, or has a high temperature or you are really worried, take the child to hospital where it can be put into an oxygen tent.

Homeopathic remedies
Give Aconite for fear, and take it yourself. Then give Spongia or Hepar Sulph.

Herbal remedy
Give 4 ml of bloodroot tincture.

DIARRHOEA

This is unusual in breast-fed babies who may normally
have several seedy, yellow, fluid stools per day. Suspect
diarrhoea if they become unusually watery, frequent or
smell different. It is more common in bottle-fed babies
because formula milk does not have the same protective
qualities as breast milk. Alternating between the two can
lead to diarrhoea by altering the pH balance in the gut.

Diarrhoea must be taken seriously in babies because
they do not have to lose much fluid to become seriously
dehydrated. This is indicated if the baby's eyes are
sunken, the soft spot on the top of its head becomes
concave and the skin is losing its elasticity. In this case
you will be able to pinch a fold and it will take far longer
than usual to return to normal. The baby's mouth will be
dry and the urine output will be much less and the colour
dark yellow. If any of these symptoms are present, call
your doctor.

Remedies for mild diarrhoea include giving the baby a
teaspoonful of puréed carrot, giving 1 fl oz (25 ml) of the
water in which rice has been boiled, or maintaining the
balance of electrolytes by giving the baby boiled water and
Dioralyte, a salt and dextrose mixture available from
chemists. In an emergency make your own with (1/2 litre)
boiled water, 1 tablespoonful suger, honey or glucose, 1/8
teaspoon sodium bicarbonate and 1/8 teaspoon salt. A
little yarrow or meadowsweet decoction may also ease the
problem. Persistent diarrhoea can be caused by allergy
(see p. 154). Baby massage can help.

Diarrhoea can cause awful nappy rash, so be sure to
change the nappy as soon as it is dirtied, and put lots of
cream on to protect the skin from acid stools.

Toddler diarrhoea, known as peas and carrots
syndrome, results in chronic diarrhoea with the food
passing through the child only partially-digested, and
often follows an attack of gastro-enteritis. Small doses of
Prime-dophulus a milk-free form of lacto bacillus, may
help.

Homeopathic remedies

Give ABC at the start. For diarrhoea with or without
vomiting, from food that was bad or too much fruit — give
Arsen Alb every two hours. If it persists consult a
homeopath. For painless diarrhoea give Acid Phos. For
green slimy stools during teething — give Chamomilla.

EAR INFECTIONS

A cold can lead to an infection of the middle ear which
causes the eardrum to bulge out painfully. Although the
cause may not be immediately apparent, you will know
that something is wrong if your baby has earache, because
it is likely to cry a lot, put its hand to its ear if old enough
and may develop a temperature. If it is left untreated, the
pus will eventually build up so that the eardrum bursts
and the pus drains out. Although the ear drum is likely to
heal satisfactorily, many doctors prefer to treat the
condition with antibiotics because there is a slight risk of
the infection spreading and because they will eventually
stop the pain. Some children suffer repeatedly from ear
infections and can be helped by treatment from a cranial
osteopath or a homeopath.

Maggie Tisserand suggests putting one drop of lavender
oil on cotton wool and putting it in the child's outer ear
to ease the pain.

David Hoffman in *The Holistic Herbal* suggests the
juice of pennywort leaves, put into the ear canal and
plugged with cotton wool. Mullein oil or Lobelia tincture
can be used in the same way instead.

Homeopathic remedies

Give ABC at the first sign of earache. If the child is
changeable, pathetic and not thirsty, give Pulsatilla 30. If
the earache is throbbing and the child is feverish, give
Belladonna 30. Repeat the treatment frequently, as often
as every 15 minutes, until there is an improvement. If
there is not a prompt response call your homeopath or
doctor.

ECZEMA

This is a condition where the skin comes up in red spots
which coalesce into smooth orangey flat patches. These
patches often itch intensely. If it is scratched, the skin
starts to weep and become rough and cracked. Eczema
commonly starts in the crooks of the knees and elbows, on
the cheeks and behind the ears.

Eczema is often an allergic response, frequently to cow's
milk (see p. 154) or to something that the skin has come
in contact with. This might be the washing powder or
conditioner that the child's sheets or clothes have been
washed in. Try using a pure soap powder and giving an
extra rinse. Boots make a conditioner especially for
sensitive skins. Wool often provokes eczema, so use a
duvet instead of blankets and cover a sheepskin with a
sheet. Buy cotton underclothes if possible as cotton is best
next to the skin.

Children with eczema are thought to be deficient in
gamma-linolenic acid. They can be helped by giving
Efamol — start with 500 mg daily and increase until the
eczema is improved.

Dry skin may be helped by applying very dilute Rose oil
in an almond oil base.

Eczema may also be helped by applying breast milk to
the skin, putting bran or oatmeal in the baby's bath, or by
applying Dandelion juice, Nelson's hypercal ointment or
Rumex ointment. Avoid using soap on the damaged skin.
Fluid extract of goldenseal stings on contact and stains
the skin yellow temporarily, but is very effective in
stopping the itching and healing the condition. Eczema
may require constitutional treatment from a homeopath.

FEVERS

Fevers are common in early childhood, with some children
seeming to be more susceptible than others, although most
get them with the infectious diseases. Sometimes children

have a raised temperature for 24 hours for no obvious reason. It is usually highest in the evening and lowest in the morning.

A child with a temperature will have a hot head, cold hands and feet and may be flushed. As the temperature rises they will either become drowsy or fretful depending on the reason for the fever. A baby with a high temperature will be hot all over and feel like a little hot water bottle. The higher the temperature the more likely that the child will tolerate a thermometer under its arm. You should get a young baby with a temperature checked by your doctor; as he or she grows you will feel better able to cope with a fever by yourself.

A fever is not necessarily a bad thing, it helps to burn off the infection and shorten the illness. Paracetamol elixir is useful to bring down a temperature that is going too high or to ease pain, but it is best if possible to let the child sleep it off. They may want to sleep all day and night, and be off their food and drink, although they should be offered drinks frequently.

Make sure that a child with a fever is lightly clad — a vest and nappy may be enough. If the temperature goes above 103°F (40°C), you may need to take steps to bring it down. This can be done by sponging the child with luke-warm water and allowing it to dry naturally. The cooling efect can be enhanced by adding either vinegar or Lavender oil to the water. You can also try wrapping the feet in compresses soaked in cold water to which two drops of Eucalyptus oil have been added. In extreme cases you may need to use a fan as well. Some children have febrile convulsions with a high temperature — alarming fits which end in sleep. These children need to be kept cool when their temperature starts to rise.

You can bring a small child's temperature down by giving it 10 drops of echinacea tincture in 4 fl oz (120 ml) of boiled water. It may help breast-fed babies if you take it yourself. Garlic perles squirted into the mouth or chewed if the child is old enough can be as effective as antibiotics. Give a minimum of six per day.

A homeopathic remedy is to give ABC every 15 minutes until there is an improvement.

HEART MASSAGE

Use if the heartbeat is less than 60 per minute (or one a second). Depress the breastbone by 2 cm twice per second, and give a mouthful of air every fourth compression. Use fingertip pressure for babies, and the heel of one hand for children. Continue until the baby improves or help arrives.

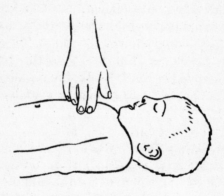

Heart massage

NAPPY RASH

Most babies get nappy rash at some time. It is easier to prevent than to cure. It starts for all sorts of reasons, including a reaction to something on the skin — this may be anything from the lotion, soap and water, cream, disposable wipes or even the nappy. If you are using terries the baby can be sensitive to the washing powder, conditioner or nappy cleanser. Use a pure soap washing powder and cut out the conditioner, and put them through an extra rinse cycle. Some mothers find that changing the brand of disposable nappy cures nappy rash.

Nappy rash is sometimes caused by teething or by food the child has eaten — fruit juice, for instance often causes a rash. To cope with it, change the nappy more frequently and use one of the healing ointments, such as calendula, hypercal, chickweed or comfrey. Nelson's ointment for burns may help and you can try mixing up a paste of goldenseal and slippery elm bark powder with water and putting it on to the skin. If possible leave the nappy off altogether or put on over-sized nappies so that the air can get to the baby's bottom.

If the nappy rash forms in patches or islands it may be caused by thrush. Treat this with an anti-fungal cream from the doctor, or make an ointment by adding a handful of the herb thuja to 7 oz (200 g) of Vaseline, simmering it for 10 minutes, then straining it through fine gauze, pressing out the liquid. Pour into a container and seal.

You may find that lightly whipping egg white and dabbing it onto the skin at change time for 24 hours may clear the rash up.

Homeopathic remedies
Give a combination of the three tissue salts Nat Phos, Nat Sulph and Silica to correct any acid or alkaline imbalance. Where the skin is red, very hot and flaky, give Arsen Alb.

RESUSCITATION

Give the baby gentle mouth-to-mouth resuscitation by lying it on a flat surface, tilting its head back and sealing the mouth *and* nose with your mouth. Puff air gently into the baby's lungs until the chest rises. Try to get in 25 breaths per minute. Continue until the baby improves or help arrives.

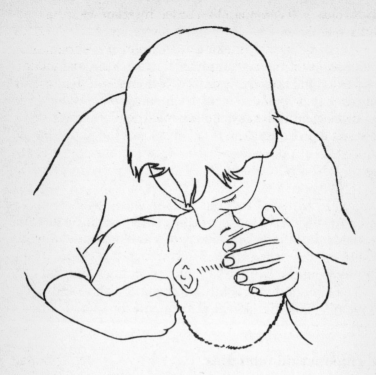

Resuscitation

STICKY EYE

Babies seem prone to a condition known as sticky eye, in which the white of the eye becomes pink and pus exudes from the corners. Either one eye or both can become infected.

Breast-milk squirted into the eye works wonderfully. Alternatively you could try bathing the eye with a weak salt solution, made up of 1 teaspoonful of salt to 1/2 a pint (300 ml) of cooled boiled water. Using a fresh piece each time, dip cotton wool into the solution and wipe gently from the inner eye outwards. Repeat a number of times during the day.

The homeopathic remedies are Pulsatilla, Arg Nit and

Nat Phos — try them in that order, together with the breast-milk.

You could also try making an infusion of eyebright or chamomile, straining it through a coffee filter, and using the liquid to bathe the eyes. Or use dilute, cold tea (colour of pine).

If the condition has not cleared within three days consult a practitioner.

SUNBURN

Take great care that babies do not get sunburn, as their tender skin can burn in a very short time. If your baby's skin is burnt use Nelson's AfterSun cream or apply their ointment for burns.

SURGERY (BABIES)

It can be a horrible experience to have your child operated on. It is always worth asking an alternative practitioner whether there is any way of remedying the complaint without surgery; for example, a child with frequent ear infection may not need to have grommets inserted into the ear drum if it is treated with cranial osteopathy to improve drainage of fluid from the inner ear.

If surgery is unavoidable, the following homeopathic remedies are advocated by Jane Arnold of the Active Birth Movement in her booklet *Homeopathy for Pregnancy, Childbirth and Infancy*.

If there is a tendency to bleed, give Phosphurus before surgery. For cut nerve endings, give Hypericum. For fear (yours or the childs), give Aconite, one dose before and one after surgery, followed by Arnica and Hypericum alternately, two doses of each, every day for several days. You may want to consult a homeopath about an antidote to a general anaesthetic.

TANTRUMS AND IRRITABILITY

Children in a really bad mood can be cheered up by being placed in a bath with a drop or two of clary sage oil in it. They may also be soothed and calmed by a gentle back massage. Massaging your child can help relieve the feeling of frustration you may feel at dealing with a child that seems determined to be unreasonable.

TEETHING

Teething is notorious for upsetting babies. There is a wide variation in the age at which the first tooth appears, and it may cause trouble long before it finally shows as a thin line in the gum. The tooth appears as a bulge under the skin and often seems to rise and recede as the gums swell in response to the small sharp edge being forced through them. It is this stage which seems to cause the most pain. Each child varies, but the teething process can be accompanied by lots of crying and fretfulness, red cheeks, night waking and dribbling. In some cases it results in diarrhoea and nappy rash and even apparent coughs and colds. It should not raise the temperature, but if your baby has a fever too, take the child to your doctor.

Water-filled teethers or rubber teething rings will help those babies who become frantic to bite on things. Others, however, cannot bear anything to touch the gums and may need paracetamol elixir to help with the pain. Nelson's make a special preparation of chamomilla granules for teething suitable for a baby that is angry, crying, who screams if he or she is put down and who has green diarrhoea.

A teething baby may be soothed by a drop of lavender or chamomile oil put onto the sheet near its head.

Homeopathic remedies
Try ABC to start, if necessary followed by one of the following remedies. For teething which results in a fever with one cheek that is especially pale or bright red, give

Aconite. For a baby that is flushed, especially if there is a tendency to convulsions, give Belladonna. For teething which makes the baby weepy, whingey and changeable, give Pulsatilla. Also try Rescue Remedy, both for yourselves and the baby. Rubbing the gums with ice, brandy or lemon juice may help ease the pain.

THRUSH

Babies sometimes get thrush inside their mouths. It shows as stubborn white patches on the cheeks. They can be removed by squirting the liquid from neo-garlic perles on to the affected parts. A homeopathic remedy is to give Borax or Candida.

Thrush also appears on the bottom as a distinctive form of nappy rash which develops in islands. This can be treated topically (see p. 171) and also systemically, by giving the child 2 garlic perles three times a day, until it clears.

Recurrent thrush may mean that you should consider treatment from a homeopath.

VOMITING

Babies are often a little bit sick — and a little goes a long way. Some babies seem to enjoy feeding and then sending the surplus back, while seeming quite happy and gaining weight. Some are decidely more prone to posseting in this way than others. It creates a lot of mess and washing, but there is nothing wrong with the baby. You can prevent your child being a sicky baby by acupuncture treatments at 14 and 26 weeks of pregnancy. Be aware of the possibility of food intolerance causing vomiting when you start weaning.

There are two kinds of vomiting which should be taken seriously. The first is due to infection, when a baby suddenly and repeatedly vomits large amounts. It may be unable to keep anything down and may well have diarrhoea as well. Give Dioralyte to drink (see p. 166) and seek help if the baby vomits more than two complete feeds consecutively. Meadowsweet infusion can help to settle the stomach.

The other type of serious vomiting is due to pyloric stenosis. This either starts suddenly or builds up gradually, and consists of the baby vomiting following feeds in such a way that vomit shoots out of the mouth and lands some feet away; it is known as projectile vomiting. It is most common in boys and it generally starts after three weeks. Treatment is essential either by operation or from a cranial osteopath.

USEFUL
ADDRESSES

Council for Complementary and Alternative Medicine
Suite One, 19A Cavendish Square, London W1M 9AD.
01-409-1440

ACUPUNCTURE

The British Acupuncture Association and Register
34 Alderney Street, London SW1. 01-834-1012

Will supply a register of acupuncturists and a handbook
in return for £1.50.

Acumedic Centre East Asia Co. Ltd
103 Camden High Street, London NW1. 01-388-5783

Shop selling books about acupuncture, moxa, needles, etc.

BACH FLOWER REMEDIES

Dr Edward Bach Centre
Mount Vernon, Wallingford, Oxon, OX10 0PZ

Supplies a booklet, *The Twelve Healers*, for 50p.

CHIROPRACTIC

British Chiropractic Association
Premier House, 10 Greycoat Place, London SW1P 1SB.
01-222-8866

Will supply a list of qualified chiropractors if you send a
9″ × 6″ SAE and two first-class stamps.

HOMEOPATHY

The British Homeopathic Association
27a Devonshire Street, London W1N 1RJ. 01-935-2163

Will supply a list of medically qualified doctors who are also qualified in homeopathy and pharmacists stocking homeopathic medicines.

The Society of Homeopaths
11a Bampton Street, Tiverton, Devon EX16 6HH

Will supply a list of registered homeopaths.

There are six NHS homeopathic hospitals to which you can be referred by your doctor:

The Bristol Homeopathic Hospital
Cotham Road, Bristol BS6 6JU

The Glasgow Homeopathic Hospital
1000 Great Western Road, Glasgow G12 0NR

The Liverpool Homeopathic Clinic
The Department of Homeopathic Medicine, The Mossley Hill Hospital, Park Road, Liverpool L18

The Manchester Homeopathic Clinic
Brunswick Street, Manchester M13 9ST

The Royal London Homeopathic Hospital
Great Ormond Street, London WC1 3HR

The Tunbridge Wells Homeopathic Hospital
Church Road, Tunbridge Wells, Kent

HYPNOTHERAPY

British Hypnotherapy Association
67 Upper Berkely Street, London W1H 7DH. 01-723-4443

British Society of Medical and Dental Hypnosis
42 Links Road, Ashstead, Surrey KT21 2HJ. 03722 73522

MEDICAL HERBALISM

The National Institute of Medical Herbalists
34 Cambridge Road, London SW7. 01-228-4417

OSTEOPATHY

The General Council and Register of Osteopaths
1 Suffolk Street, London SW1Y 4HG. 01-839-2060

Will supply a list of registered osteopaths for £1.40.

CRANIAL OSTEOPATHY

Sutherland Society
5 Weston Avenue, Mount Hooton Road, Nottingham NG7
4BA. 0602 785533

REBIRTHING

Rebirth Society
18a Great Percy Street, London WC1 9QP. 01-833-0741

WOMEN'S HEALTH

Women's Natural Health Centre
169 Malden Road, London NW5. 01-267-5301

Healing, osteopathy, touch for health, homeopathy. (For
women on low incomes, maximum fee £6.00.)

Women's Health Information Centre
52/54 Featherstone Street, London EC1. 01-251-6580

SUPPLIERS OF HERBS AND ESSENTIAL OILS BY POST

G. Baldwin and Co.
171/173 Walworth Road, London SE17 1RW.
01-703-5550

Cathay of Bournemouth Ltd
32 Cleveland Road, Bournemouth, Dorset. 0202-37178

Gerard House
736 Christchurch Road, Bournemouth, Dorset.
0202-35352

Also sells tissue salts.

Neal's Yard Apothecary
2 Neal's Yard, Covent Garden, London WC2

Also supplies homeopathic remedies — reasonably priced.

D. Napier and Sons Ltd
17/18 Bristo Place, Edinburgh, Scotland

Self-Heal Herbs
Hayes Corner, South Cheriton, Templecombe, Somerset.
0963 70300

Butterbur and Sage Ltd
PO Box 41, Southall, Middlesex UB1 3BZ

Supplies essential oils only.

The number of chemists who stock homeopathic preparations is increasing all the time. You can get a list of those in your area if you send a stamped addressed envelope to the British Homeopathic Association (address above). The following are **homeopathic pharmacies** which stock all the remedies and will supply them by mail order. They will advise personal callers, and have a telephone/postal service. Tell them if it is urgent.

Ainsworths
38 New Cavendish Street, London W1M 7LH.
01-935-5330

Galen Pharmacy
1 South Terrace, South Street, Dorchester, Dorset.
0305 3996

Helios Homeopathic Pharmacy
92 Camden Road, Tunbridge Wells, Kent TN1 2QP.
0892 36393

A. Nelson and Co. Ltd
73 Duke Street, London W1. 01-946-8527

Weleda (UK) Ltd
Heanor Road, Ilkeston, Derbyshire DE7 8DR.
0602 303151

Action for Victims of Medical Accidents
135, Stockwell Road, London SW9. 01-737-2434

Active Birth Movement
55 Dartmouth Park Road, London NW5. 01-267-3006

Association for the Improvement in Maternity Services
163 Liverpool Road, London N1 0RF. 01-278-5628

Association of Breastfeeding Mothers
10 Herschell Road, London SE23 1EN

Association for Post-Natal Illness
Queen Charlotte's Hospital
Goldhawk Road, London W6. 01-741-5019

Association of Radical Midwives
62 Greetsby Hill, Ormskirk, Lancashire L39 2DT.
0695 72776. 01-580-2991

Asthma Society
300 Upper Street, London N1 2XX. 01-226-2260

Baby Soother Tape
JayGee Cassettes
10 Golf Links Road, Burnham-on-Sea, Somerset TA8
2PW

Cry-sis
BM Crysis
London WC1N 3XX. 01-404-5011

Down's Children's Association
12-13 Clapham Common South Side, London SW4 7AA.
01-720-0008

Ergo Computer Accessories (advice on dangers of
VDU screens)
Prospect House, 44-52 Oxford Rd, Reading, Berks. 0734
596338

Foresight (pre-conceptual care)
The Old Vicarage, Church Lane, Witley, Goldalming,
Surrey GU8 5PN. 042879 4500

The Foundation for the Study of Infant Deaths
15 Belgrave Square, London SW1X 7HD. 01-235
1721. 01-245-9421

Gingerbread (single parents)
35 Wellington Street, London WC2E 7BN. 01-240-0953

Health Rights Project
157 Waterloo Road, London SE1. 01-928-0080

La Leche League (breastfeeding advice)
Box 3424, London WC1 6XX. 01-404-5011

London Hazards Centre (advise on chemical risks to pregnancy)
103 Borough Road, London SE1. 01-261-9558

Lullababy (baby soothing tape)
Highview, Kings Thorn, Hertford HR2 8BR. 0981-540 288

MAMA (Meet-a-Mum Association)
3 Woodside Ave, London SE25. 01-654-3137

Maternity Alliance
15 Britannia Street, London WC1X 9JP. 01-837-1265

Maternity Defence Fund
33 Castle Street, Henley-in-Arden, Warwickshire

Miscarriage Association
18 Stoneybrook Close, West Bretton, Wakefield WF4 4TP, West Yorkshire. 0924 85515

National Association for the Childless
318 Summer Lane, Birmingham B19 3RL. 021-359-4887

National Association for the Welfare of Children in Hospital
Argyle House, 29-31 Euston Road, London NW1. 01-833-2041

National Caesarean Support Network
c/o Sheila Tunstall, 2 Hurst Park Drive, Huyton, Liverpool L36 1TF

National Childbirth Trust
Alexandra House, Oldham Terrace, Acton, London W3 6NH. 01-992-8637

National Child Minding Association
204/206 High Street, Bromley, Kent BR1 1PP. 01-464-6164

National Council for One Parent Families
255 Kentish Town Road, London NW5 2LX. 01-267-1361

National Eczema Society
Tavistock House North, Tavistock Square, London WC1.
01-388-4097

Neen Pain Management Systems (TNS)
The Pharmacy Store, Church St, East Dereham, Norfolk
NR19 1DJ. 0362 698966

Nippers (National Information for Prematures —
Education, Resources and Support)
c/o The Sam Segal Perinatal Unit, St Mary's Hospital,
Praed Street, Paddington, London W2 1NY. 01-725-1487

Novafon Ltd
2 Atholl Rd, Pitlochry PH16 5BX. 0796 2735

Parents Anonymous
6 Manor Gardens, London N7 6LA. 01-263-8918

Pre-Eclamptic Toxaemia Society
33 Keswick Ave, Hullbridge, Essex SS5 6JL. 0702-231689

Barbara Pickard (advice on morning sickness)
Lane End Farm, Denton, Ilkley, West Yorkshire LS29
0HP. 0943-609209

Pregnancy Advisory Service
11-13 Charlotte Street, London W1P 1HD. 01-637-8962

Relaxation for Living (relaxation techniques)
29 Burwood Park Road, Walton-on-Thames, Surrey

Royal College of Midwives
15 Mansfield Street, London W1M 0BE. 01-580-6523/4/5

Support After Termination for Abnormality
22 Upper Woburn Place, London WC1H 0CP

Stillbirths and Neonatal Deaths Society
28 Portland Place, London W1N 4DE. 01-436-5881

Society to Support Home Confinements
Lydgate, Lydgate Lane, Wolsingham, Bishop Auckland,
Co. Durham DL13 3HN. 0388 528044

Twins and Multiple Birth Association
54 Broad Lane, Hampton, Middlesex. 01-941-0641

West London Birth Centre
33 Colebrooke Avenue, Ealing, London W13 8JZ.
01-997-5275 or 01-568-0371

Women and Work Hazards Group
British Society for Social Responsibility in Science, 9
Poland Street, London W1. 01-437-2728

Women's Health Information Centre
52-54 Featherstone Street, London EC1.
01-251-6580

Working Mothers' Association
7 Spencer Walk, London SW15 1PL. 01-788-2565

RECOMMENDED READING

General
Lucienne Lanson, *From Woman to Woman*, Penguin, 1983
Dr Caroline Shreeve, *Alternative Dictionary of Symptoms and Cures*, Century, 1986
Nicky Wesson, *The Assertive Pregnancy*, Thorsons, 1988
Patsy Westcott, *Alternative Health Care*, Thorsons, 1987

Homeopathy
Drs Sheila and Robin Gibson, *Homeopathy for Everyone*, Penguin, 1987

Medical herbalism
Juliette de Bairacli Levy, *The Illustrated Herbal Handbook*, Faber, 1982
David Hoffman, *The Holistic Herbal*, Findhorn Press, 1983
Anne McIntyre, *Herbs for Pregnancy and Childbirth*, Sheldon Press, 1988
Michael McIntyre, *Herbalism for Everyone*, Penguin, 1988
Susun Weed, *The Wise Woman Herbal for the Childbearing Year*, Ash Tree Publishing, USA, 1985, available from Compendium Books, 234 Camden High Street, London NW1 8QS

Aromatherapy
Maggie Tisserand, *Aromatherapy for Women*, Thorsons, 1985

Diet in pregnancy
Catherine Lewis, *Good Food before Birth*, Unwin Hyman, 1984

Massage
Clare Maxwell Hudson, *The Complete Book of Massage*, Dorling Kindersley, 1988
Stephen Russell and Yehudi Gordon, *Massage for Life*, available by post from 156 Hendon Way, London NW2 0NE at £3.40, including postage and packing.

Acupuncture
Julian Kenyon, *Acupressure Techniques*, Thorsons, 1987
Dr Ruth Lever, *Acupuncture For Everyone*, Penguin, 1987

INDEX

Page numbers in *italics* refer to illustrations.

INDEX

cramp, 52, *53*
cranial osteopathy: 3, 8–10; and colic, 161; and depression, 126; and infertility, 25–6; and the placenta, 123
croup, 165
cystitus, 54–5

decoctions, 13
depression, 124–7
diarrhoea, 84, 166–7
diet, 33–4
diphtheria, 153
doctor, when to call, 149–50
'doulas' (birth companions), 40
duct-mastitis (blocked milk ducts), 136–7

ear infections, 167
eczema, 168
endometriosis, 24
engorgement, 135
environmental hazards, 20
epidural anaesthesia, 93–4
episiotomy, 101–3
exercises, 37–9

fainting, 55–6
fear, 56–7
fertility cycle, 27
fetal distress, 114
fevers, 168–70
first aid, 150
fluid extracts, 14
forceps delivery, 104–5, 115
forgetfulness, 58

German measles, 20, 151

haemorrhage, 112–13
haemorrhoids (piles), 58–9
Hahnemann, Samuel, 10
headaches, 60–1
heartburn, 61
Heimlich manoeuvre, *157*

herbal remedies: and breast feeding, 133; and colic, 161; and constipation, 52; and cramp, 54; and croup, 165; and cystitus, 55; and episiotomy, 103; and exhaustion in labour, 109; and haemorrhage, 113; and headaches, 60; and heartburn, 61–2; and hypertension, 64; and insomnia, 66; and labour, 95; and miscarriage, 68, 71; and morning sickness, 72; and piles, 59; and the placenta, 123; and slow labour, 106
herbalism, 12–14
herbs, to be avoided in pregnancy, 13
herpes, 63, 114
homeopathic remedies: 3, 10–12; and cystitis, 55; and anaemia, 42; and backache, 43–5; and bleeding in pregnancy, 46; and breast feeding, 132, 133, 137; and breech babies, 49; and caesarean section, 116; and chest infections, 150; and colic, 162; and constipation, 163; and cramp, 54; and croup, 165; and depression, 126; and diarrhoea, 167; and ear infections, 167; and episiotomy, 103; and exhaustion in labour, 109; and fainting, 56; and fear, 57; and haemorrhage, 113; and hypertension, 65; and infertility, 25; and insomnia, 66; and miscarriage, 69, 71; and morning sickness, 72–3; and nappy rash, 171; and the placenta, 122, 124; and premature babies, 76; and slow labour, 107; and varicose veins, 82; and colds, 159; and constipation, 51; and heartburn, 62; and piles, 59;

ABOUT THE AUTHOR

NICKY WESSON became a postnatal supporter for the National Childbirth Trust following the birth of her first child. She is currently training to be an NCT antenatal teacher.

Since the first publication of her first book, *The Assertive Pregnancy* (Thorsons), she has become convinced of the superiority of alternative approaches to medicine, and is now a member of the Association for the Improvement in Maternity Services. Optima will be publishing her next book *Home Birth* in 1989. She lives in Middlesex with her husband and four children.

All Optima books are available at your bookshop or newsagent, or can be ordered from the following address:

Optima, Cash Sales Department,
PO Box 11, Falmouth, Cornwall TR10 9EN

Please send cheque or postal order (no currency), and allow 60p for postage and packing for the first book, plus 25p for the second book and 15p for each additional book ordered up to a maximum charge of £1.90 in the UK.

Customers in Eire and BFPO please allow 60p for the first book, 25p for the second book plus 15p per copy for the next 7 books, thereafter 9p per book.

Overseas customers please allow £1.25 for postage and packing for the first book and 28p per copy for each additional book.